By Sword or by Hailstone

God's Plan for Victory

Gina Routon

Dedication

To the *valiant* one, who stands in the
presence of God, who sees his enemies trodden down.

*Give us help from trouble; for vain is the help of man. Through God we shall
do valiantly; for he it is that shall tread down our enemies.*
—Psalm 108:12–13

Preface

I have not considered myself a writer but by writing this book I hope to tell my story. A story that I hope will encourage the reader and testify of the great hope that we have in Christ. The undeniable power of His Word, His steadfast and unchangeable character, and unfathomable love that He has for us, His children.

This is the story of how my life changed forever in the summer of 2014. When the mundane became the precious. When all that I had been taught was put to the test. This is a story of how I learned to rest in the deep water and find strength for living each day. This is the story of God's miraculous sustaining power.

If you've chosen to pick this book up to read for yourself or to share with a friend, I pray that you see Christ in the pages, that you will find strength for your own journey, and that you will discover an inexhaustible power supply in the name above all names, Jesus, the Son of God. The challenge, the battle, the wins and losses. Through it all He never leaves us. All things are possible to him who believes.

Contents

Acknowledgments

To my forever love, Kurt Mathew. You've always been the one. Your confidence in me has been my occasion to soar. Thank you for believing in me.

To my beautiful, ever-expanding family. I'm so glad God allowed me to be your mom. Your faith has made you a force to be reckoned with. I see strength and courage; I see love.

To my mom and dad, DC and Virginia. The roots you've given me were my strength when the storm came. You are a testament to God's goodness in the land of the living.

To the body of Christ, my church family, thank you for shaking heaven for me.

To those of you who said, "Write a book," and to the one who said, "Write it, and I will help you make it happen." You know who you are. Thank you for encouraging me to put this testimony to pen. May God bless you richly.

Chapter 1
FAITH SHAKEN

As July came to a close, August was signaling the end of a busy summer. Life alongside my husband, Kurt, in full-time pastoral ministry had been blissfully busy. We both enjoyed life and living it to the fullest. As well as being pastors, we worked jobs outside of the church and enjoyed spending days off with our children and grandchildren. This particular summer we had also managed a firework stand for several weeks around the holiday. But as I looked on my schedule and realized I was running out of summer days, I knew I would need to get whatever I was going to do done before the school year began. My teenage daughter, Zoe, was needing one last summer trip, and as my parents' only daughter, I was needing to go home for a visit. So I made the decision to make the time. Kurt's job responsibilities would not allow him to make the trip with us, so Zoe and I packed up the car, said good-bye to Kurt, and headed from our home in Missouri to my hometown of Paris, Texas. We were looking forward to a fun mother-daughter three-day trip.

The first day was perfect for traveling—sunny, clear, and no sign of any troubles. We made good time, and in just under six hours, we crossed the Red River Bridge that marked the Texas state line and took the extra time to stop and make a memory by taking our picture by the state of Texas granite marker. We arrived at my parents' home not long after. Mom and Dad were waiting.

There is something about the familiarity of coming home that brings comfort to the soul. For me it's a place of welcome, a place to be yourself. It fits—no worries, just breathing in the Texas summer air and feeling the warm sun on my face, leaving behind work and daily responsibilities to rest and relax. I was looking forward to the next few days with family, just enjoying some much-needed downtime.

It was good to see my mom and dad, who are both in their late seventies and a testimony to God's keeping power. We hugged, greeted each other, and began making plans for the next few days. Shopping and eating at our favorite restaurants were of course at the top of the to-do list. We didn't want to waste any precious time.

We stayed up late that first night just catching up and enjoying one another.

The following morning I woke early with a sharp pain in my upper right abdomen. It was not what I was expecting and certainly not part of the plan. I had been hoping to sleep in and have the luxury of being lazy, but the pain was not allowing it. I tried adjusting myself to different positions, but nothing really helped. When I got out of bed, it was even harder to stand up straight. I walked around the room for a bit hoping it would pass. It was not. After some time I decided it warranted telling my mom.

So I went to her dressing area where she was getting ready for the day. I told her how I was hurting.

"Maybe it was just trapped gas?" she questioned.

But several antacids later, I said decidedly it was not anything of the like. We had to cancel our dinner plans that evening, and I began to wonder if I would even be able to make the drive back to Missouri. My trip home, our plans for fun and relaxation, had turned into something very different. Why was this happening? I could not figure out what could be wrong.

The third day came, and I still was not better. I was becoming conscious of the discomfort with every breath as it hurt when I took in a deep breath. I found that I could lie on my left side and have some relief. I called my husband and told him he may have to come and get me if something did not change. We were all praying.

The fourth day came, and it was time to head home. I was feeling some relief. The pain was less but nagging. I did, however, feel that I could make the drive home. This trip had not been what I had hoped for, but a least we got to visit with family.

I arrived back home in Missouri, and life resumed as normal. The pain had subsided and was almost undetectable. I had a bout with allergies before the trip and had some coughing. In an attempt to explain my pain away, I thought possibly I had displaced a rib during a coughing episode. I had heard of that sort of thing happening. So I went on. After all I had always been healthy. I was rarely sick with anything and had no real health issues.

But on my fourth day back home from Texas, the pain was back with a vengeance. It was August 22, three days before my forty-seventh birthday. Kurt and Zoe were out buying my birthday cards when I called him on his cell phone to let him know I thought I would have to go to the ER. The pain was worse. He finished up with his card shopping and came home to find me lying on my left side in the bed. I could barely roll out of bed, it was such an excruciating pain. He helped me to the car, and we were on our way. We really had no idea.

We waited five hours in the ER just to be seen. By the time I was called back, the pain had eased again. I told them my rib theory. I don't think they were buying that one. They started with blood work, checked to make sure it was not my heart, and proceeded with the standard chest X-ray. It was now ten o'clock at night. I lay there waiting.

I was fully expecting them to find nothing. Surely whatever this was would be simple with an easy explanation. The doctor returned to my bedside and said the blood work was abnormal and might indicate I had a blood clot.

"What?" That was my first thought—what? "What do you mean a blood clot?" I was shocked he even said it.

However, before the night was over, there would be many more expressions of unbelievable, even unspeakable words, words that my husband would say left you feeling discombobulated.

So we waited. I lay there in the ER bed, Kurt by my side and my precious Zoe sitting in a chair leaned against a wall. I was concerned that she probably needed to get home. I wished we could just all go home. I wished this wasn't happening. It seemed so surreal.

He saw something. Yes, those were the ER doctor's next words to us when he returned to my room.

I was thinking to myself, "Hmm, what does he mean he saw something?"

A partial of something showed up in the chest X-ray, he explained. The X-ray had caught a glimpse of the top of something on my liver. And my liver enzymes were elevated.

Here we went again, my mind whirling around trying to understand what was being said. The words that were about to come would completely blindside my husband and me. These were words that would shake us to the core.

When we asked what it could be, the doctor said without hesitation, "It is either a cluster of blood vessels"—nothing to worry about—"or it is cancer."

And that was how he said it—just that plainly.

My mind went everywhere in an instant. For a moment I didn't think I would be able to breathe. I wanted to run. And all this was said in front of my thirteen-year-old daughter. I felt as if the ceiling was closing in on me. There was an atmosphere of urgency around me as the doctor said he had ordered a CT scan and I would be staying overnight. He explained that the following morning he would be scheduling an early-morning MRI, a stress test, and possibly a liver biopsy. But for now they were going to admit me to the hospital and take me to a room. It was two o'clock in the morning. And although Kurt did not want to leave my side, I convinced him I would be all right until morning. It was best for Zoe if he take her on home and give her some normality. We held hands tightly as we said our good-bye. A million thoughts were swirling in my mind. I didn't want to let go as I felt uncertainty grip my heart. I was thinking I was not very good at being brave.

The lights were dim in the overnight room they rolled me into. The nurses were kind in an uneasy way, or that was how I perceived it. They left me there to sleep, but I reached for my phone—not to make a call but to open my Bible app and read the Word. I needed Him, the One. I needed the rock that David wrote about in Psalm 61. I was so shook I couldn't think of where to read. I had been studying the book of Isaiah during my devotion time at home, so I tried to remember what chapter I was in. I thought it was somewhere around Isaiah 37, so I typed in the thirty-seventh chapter. My eyes fell straight to verse six. It was not the chapter I had been reading; however, it was the voice of my beautiful Jesus reaching out to me in my overwhelming despair and gripping fear: "And Isaiah said unto them, 'Thus shall ye say unto your master, Thus saith the LORD: Be not afraid of the words that thou hast heard, wherewith the servants of the king of Assyria have blasphemed me.'"

Be not afraid. Those were *His* words to me in those dark, early-morning hours. I grasped the words tightly. I gulped back tears and refused to give in to utter despair. It was His Word, and His Word was truth. I clung to those words as I closed my eyes to get some rest. I won't say it was sound, but my panic had eased.

Chapter 2

WAKING UP

The next morning my eyes opened, and I had to face that this had *not* all been a bad dream, but, oh, how I wished that it had been. A nurse came in early to escort me to my very first MRI. They gave me something by mouth to relax me because I was not extremely fond of closed in spaces. OK, it did make me feel a little less stressed, but let's face it—the monster was still in the room. However, my God was in the room also. And though I heard the taunts of the enemy, the still small voice of my Father God was there whispering, "Do not be afraid."

A couple hours later, I went for a stress test. They basically just wanted to rule out any problems with my heart before they moved forward. The stress test was pretty simple. I aced it with no problem.

I was not really surprised that my stress test came back so well because I had always been pretty active. Up to this point, I would describe my lifestyle as moderately active. I had enjoyed staying healthy by routinely walking and running and was even hoping to enter my first 5K in the fall; it was on my bucket list anyway. Just seven months prior, I had surprised my husband with a vacation to Estes Park Colorado for his fiftieth birthday. We had enjoyed hiking in the Rockies.

I'm taking time to share this because I want to make a point that I did not feel sick. No big signs said anything was medically wrong with me.

That day at the hospital during the stress test, the nurses and doctor who came alongside me kept making remarks about how well I looked. I did not look sick in any way. Surely it was just a cluster of veins or something else. But by all the indicators, it was not sounding like the case. The doctor who was assigned to me that day (I did not have a family physician) did not want to send me home until I had what they saw in my liver biopsied. This in retrospect was one of the many I believe divinely orchestrated decisions the medical staff, who took such good care of me, made. So fairly quickly I was being whisked away to another apart of the hospital. Kurt had taken off work to be with me and sat beside me holding my hand and reassuring me that everything would be OK as we waited for the next doctor and the next test. This was so far away from me thinking it was just a bruised rib. Again it felt surreal, and I could not believe it was happening.

The next doctor I recall as quite an excited fellow. I would only meet him this one time. He carried an iPad in one hand and with the other reached out to shake our hands and introduce himself. He would be doing the biopsy on my liver and asked if we would like to see it, a digital picture of what he would biopsy. The next thing I knew he was whipping out the iPad and putting it in front of me.

I don't remember saying yes to wanting to see it or even if Kurt did, but the next thing I knew he was showing *them* to me—and, yes, I said *them*. He was speaking excitedly like someone who enjoyed popping a zit and he had just seen the mother of all zits and was going to get a go at it. I was not sharing in his enthusiasm. He explained that the MRI had showed not one but five tumors. This was the first time I was hearing the word *tumor*. He explained there was one really large one in the right lobe of my liver, near the top perimeter and very close to the left lobe. This undoubtedly had been the one they caught a glimpse of on the chest X-ray and most likely the culprit causing me pain. The other three tumors they called satellite tumors around the large one. I don't remember exactly where the other one was, but they were all located on the right lobe of my otherwise healthy liver. Wow, that was a lot to take in. Kurt and I just looked at one another totally stunned and speechless. Again we held hands tightly until we couldn't anymore as they rolled me to the operating room.

I woke to see my youngest son, Caleb, age twenty-four, sitting with his sister, Zoe, at the foot of my hospital bed. Kurt had to go to work for a few hours and would be back soon to pick me up. I was groggy from the drugs, and even though the mood was solemn, my beautiful children managed to make fun of my sleepy, out-of-my-head kind of talk.

I am extremely proud of all three of our children. Each one has his or her own distinct personality, as I am sure any of you with more than one child can relate. Caleb is my joyful, compassionate, yet straightforward child. I am often not sure what he is going to say at any given time, so on occasion I have held my breath and whispered prayerfully "Dear God." He looks for the good and tries to cheer me up.

He was sitting next to our youngest and only daughter, Zoe. She is our child of faith. There are ten years between her and Caleb—ten years because it took eleven years from the time God first planted the seed in our hearts to adopt from China to the day we sat in our car to hear a simple statement on the radio from Pastor Tony Evans saying if you really believed

God had spoken something to you, you would take the steps to do it. For some reason that day the light bulb went on, and we had an epiphany. Our faith without works was dead. We looked at each other surprised, as though we were hearing this concept for the first time, as though we hadn't been ministering for twenty years and hadn't preached it, oh, let's say…a million times! I'm being sarcastic here, but, really, why were we missing this?

Kurt looked at me and said, "Do you really believe God wants us to do this?"

I said unequivocally, "Yes."

He said, "So do I."

We went home that day, filled out the paper work, and sent our request in to Dillon International. It was our first faith step in bringing our daughter home. The rest is another story and another book in our journey of faith, but God made it possible, completely made it possible.

Zoe is beautiful inside and out. She wears her heart on her sleeve. She holds precious things very close, so close that sometimes it is hard for others to see. She is brave and strong.

On this day she had been holding in her tears for fear of what the ER physician had proclaimed about her mom. Her expression had been completely blank. She was putting on her brave face, that is until Caleb walked into my hospital room that day. She was sitting in a chair. She looked so alone, but then she made eye contact with her brother. He asked her if she was all right, and that was all it took. Tears came pouring. He held her close. He knew just what to say that day. And she, my sweet Zoe, was going to be OK. Her strength was going deep. God had her. He had been with her at conception when I was not. He would not fail her this day or any other day. Through all of this, her faith, along with the rest of us, our family, would be tested only to see it blossom and become a force to be reckoned with.

The doctor who had gone alongside me throughout the day came in to let me know they would be sending me home. She said she just couldn't believe it could be cancer, but if the results came back positive, they would do something. I don't think she knew what that something would be—just something. Maybe that was to make us feel better. She gave us the name of a doctor to whom they would be sending the results of the biopsy and said I would be going home shortly.

The nurse who had taken care of me through the night came in with my release papers and asked me if I went to church. I said yes.

Then she said, "If they have a prayer chain, you might want to call it and have your name put on it."

Everyone around me was seemingly feeling the gravity of the situation. I just smiled and gathered my things. It was Saturday morning, and I would have to wait until the next week to find out the results of the biopsy. I would also celebrate my forty-seventh birthday and try to absorb what had just happened. My husband would pick up the phone to break the news to my mom and dad about what we were facing. He would also have to face our three children. Our oldest two were married, so our dear daughters-in-love would also share the burden of this news. He would have to be the shoulder of strength to our precious Zoë. And as a pastor, Kurt would stand before our congregation of believers to share with them from the pulpit the battle we were facing.

I won't share his feelings here because they are his, and I won't speak to his pain in my dialogue.

Kurt was the love of my life. I had known him since we were teens in church youth group. We met at our home church in Paris, Texas, the Bonham Street Church of God. That summer of 1981, our youth pastor asked me to play the part of a Raggedy Ann in the Summer Kids Crusade. I was just entering the teen youth group and had not met all of the young people yet. The evening of the crusade, dressed in a Raggedy Ann costume, I walked into the youth pastor's office where the cast would meet before going out to perform. As I walked in the room, my eyes fixed on the handsomest smile I had ever seen. It did not matter that he was wearing a red and white polka-dotted clown costume. And, no, I don't have a thing for clowns! He had no makeup on…yet anyway. I became oblivious to the rest of the cast in the room. Everything went silent in my head; it was like momentary deafness had occurred only to me. I gave my heart away that day—love at first sight. Yeah, it's kind of corny sounding, but I'm telling you this is the way it happened for me—clown suit and all. It would take a bit longer for Kurt to feel the same way about me. But he did finally see the light and hear the music. Yes, I am laughing at this, but I am so telling the truth.

And thirty-one years later, here we are. Through our marriage we have shared much laughter and times of want and plenty. We are each other's best friends, and I am confident of this.

He has been my biggest supporter in life. Kurt believes in me, and I love him for that. He finds my goofiness appealing, and my impulsiveness he calls a sense of adventure. The man has patience! He often will quietly listen as I hatch the plan for my next Big Idea—minus the pertinent details, but nevertheless he listens. Sometimes he does so with a look that says, "What the heck are you talking about" stretched across his handsome face. But he hears me, and I love him for that too. What more could a girl want?

What we were facing on this day, however, was new territory. Kurt is my steady rock, my balance in a world of ups and downs. And although Jesus is my everything, I am grateful God has chosen to allow me to walk through life with this mighty man of valor.

We together, our family, prayed and walked through the next week one day at a time. We chose to keep this preliminary news close to home, praying and waiting.

Chapter 3
DOUBLE WHAMMY

Sitting in the doctor's office the next week, waiting for the results of the liver biopsy, I looked around and saw very few people. It was the end of the workday, and clearly I was the last patient of the day.

This is never a good sign. I have worked in healthcare before, and often we would schedule the patients receiving the bad news at the end of the day when everyone else was gone.

I looked at Kurt and told him so. We tried to smile and laugh a bit about it, trying to make light in the midst of tension. But all joking aside, we were trying to brace ourselves for the coming news and be brave.

We were finally called back. Most of the nurses were leaving, and there were no more patients to be seen anywhere. It was very quiet. The nurse seated us in a small exam room, did the necessities of taking my vitals, and then softly closed the door on her way out. The anticipation of what would come next in these moments were almost more than a soul could bare. I did not like this feeling. My primary care physician assigned to me from my ER visit came in shortly after, and again we made our introductions to another doctor and sat for the news from the biopsy. We really had no idea what we were about to hear. The doctor sat down on his rolling chair and took my chart in his hand. He began reading over it without making much eye contact with me. He explained very calmly and slowly that, yes, indeed it was cancer in my liver. Oh, those words…how could this be happening? He went on to explain the biopsy had shown colon markers.

"What?" I was not expecting that.

At this stage I was in the repeating phase. You know, the doctor says cancer, and I say, "Cancer?" He says from my colon, and I say, "Colon?"

In simple terms the cancer in my liver did not originate there; it came by way of the colon. Bam! Double whammy! I was just blown away by this news.

My husband remembers me asking bluntly, "So what are you saying? Do I have six months or a year?"

In essence I was asking in the world of cancer if this was a big deal or a little deal. I needed to see the whole picture so I could process and access properly what was happening. I had lots of questions. How would they treat it? Could they just take it out? So many questions. However, he was not going to be the one to give me the answers or the details I sought. That would be the oncologist's job—another doctor visit to yet another new face. There were steps to follow to receive the news, and his was just to tell me officially, "Yes you got it; you have cancer. Now let's make you an appointment with someone in this field of specialty."

My husband quickly asked him for a prescription for me, something for my nerves. I had never taken any medication before for this type of thing, but then again I had never faced a situation like this before.

Kurt is forever wanting to fix anything and everything for me and make things all right. I can't imagine what he must have been feeling in these moments. He wanted me not to be afraid. He was trying to help me. I did not put up a resistance to his request. Quite frankly I didn't know how I was going to handle all of this completely ridiculously sounding news at this point anyway. We did find out later, however, for me, that praise and worship music playing by the bed at night worked better than Xanax—for me anyway.

Secondly Kurt asked if we could leave town and go on a short vacation. We had planned a trip to Florida. Could we take a few days and escape? I could see him thinking about it, and then he offered a yes. He thought this would be OK. It could only be a few days though because he would be scheduling a CT scan of my abdomen and a colonoscopy, and this would need to be done as soon as they could get me in. He said he would call with the appointment times, and we would not need to miss those appointments. As the doctor was stressing the importance of this, I could see it would be a priority.

We gave the news to my family and went home to pack. We were very much on a mission; that mission at the moment was to run...run far, far away. I remember telling my husband just to get in the car and drive. I think I thought the further we could get away from the place we heard the news, the less real it would be. We loaded up the car quickly, and Kurt, Zoe, and I left town that evening. We could not get away fast enough. Florida was our plan by way of Interstate 10, allowing us to stopover in New Orleans. We had lived for a time in Louisiana. Our first pastorate was on the North Shore, a little place by the name of Folsom—great memories. We were way overdue for this trip. We had not been able to take a vacation the year before, so this was supposed to be our year to go. But in the car on the way, I started to feel uncomfortable; the familiar pain was trying to come back. I found if I laid my seat back and stretched out a bit, it wasn't so bad.

The next day we made it to New Orleans, checked into our room, and began to look forward to distraction. Zoë wanted to go to the aquarium, and I wanted to sit at Café Du Monde and have a cup of coffee and a beignet while listening to the street musicians play. The thoughts of a cancer diagnosis were never far from our minds. Try as we might to escape, it was not going away.

Meanwhile my mom and dad back in our home church were rallying the warriors—prayer warriors, that is. A tactical prayer strategy was coming into place on my behalf, the foundation of what would be my ultimate defense, the Word of God in action for me. I was too weak, wounded at this point to take my stand. An undercut from the enemy of my soul had blindsided me. I was reeling in a daze like a fighter in the ring, not knocked out but staggering. But there they were, my brothers and sisters in the Lord ready to stand in the gap for me.

I can see them in my mind's eye standing arm in arm around me, covering me with prayer, each prayer a jab to the enemy's throat, disabling his voice of lies. Other believers would join in later, but this group, my home church in Paris, Texas, was the first on the scene. Their prayers were so fervent, red hot with the anointing, waging war in the heavenlies on my behalf. They were not going to stand by and offer a sweet compassionate pat on the back; not that compassion doesn't have a place, but what I needed now was not soft and peaceable. I needed warriors willing to wield the sword of the spirit in faith on my behalf. Physically I had been diagnosed with this awful disease, and spiritually my faith was being assaulted unlike anything I had ever before experienced. Thank God I had a strong family of God to call on to unite with us in prayer.

It just so happened that the pastor of mine and Kurt's home church in Texas, where our parents still attend, was Bishop Doug Holt and his wife, Sandy. He was the youth pastor who had introduced Kurt and me thirty years earlier in that Summer Kids Crusade. Now he was the pastor of the local congregation. I don't think relationships are coincidental. Rev. Holt took my need directly to the congregation, and they in turn took my affliction and carried it as their own, lifting me up in prayer, interceding for me. Other churches, people, and dear friends from across the country came alongside me also as the news of my illness got out, but these were my first

> Confess your faults one to another, and pray one for another, that ye may be healed. *The effectual fervent prayer* of a righteous man *availeth much* (James 5:16).

responders.

That first night in our hotel room, the thoughts going through my mind were awful. I lay beside my husband and wondered how he saw me. How would he find me attractive, a woman with the tag line of death over her head? I would be the absolute opposite of alive and vivacious. That did not sound appealing to me. How would anything ever be the same again? I struggled not to see myself as the enemy saw me. I thought of my daughter. She was too young not to have a mom around. I thought of her first date, first prom, and first pair of high-heel shoes—the oh-so-important firsts that I did not want to miss. I thought of my grandchildren and unborn grandchildren. I thought of my husband and our future dreams. I thought until I did not want to think anymore. I tried to sleep that night, but I was restless.

The next morning was Sunday. I woke up and thought about the lesson I had taught my early-elementary class the previous Wednesday night at church, which was before I received the big news from the doctor on the following Friday. I taught them the lesson of David and Goliath. I shared with them how David was not afraid to face the giant who taunted the children of Israel because he stood not on his own abilities but in God's. I shared how the enemy tried to intimidate David by taunting him with words, by bullying him, by bullying God's chosen people. I talked about strength, God's strength, and the unmitigated audacity of this uncircumcised giant to defy the living God. Who did he think he was?: "Then David said to the Philistine, 'You come to me with a sword, with a spear, and with a javelin. But I come to you in the name of the LORD of hosts, the God of the armies of Israel, whom you have defied'" (1 Samuel 17:45 NKJV).

Sunday morning I was grasping hold of what I knew to be true. God was bigger than this diagnosis. God was a Big God, and I didn't like being bullied by the devil and his spirits of fear.

Kurt and Zoe got up and dressed to go downstairs for breakfast. I made the decision to stay in the room while they went down to eat. I went for my phone and turned on my Pandora app to hear some music. My faith was stirring within me, and I needed to ramp up my praise.

Now if you use Pandora, you know that you select a genre and then get what they play. On this morning the song that came on first was "God's Not Dead" by the Newsboys. Let me tell you, I got my praise on that morning. I danced and did what I call my war dance while singing very loudly, "God's not dead. He's surely alive. He's living on the inside roaring like a lion." I could hear my Jesus. I could see Him as the lion of the tribe of Judah, and He was roaring. My Jesus was alive and well! My faith was rising up.

Praise is so very important. I had the joy of discovering the power of praise early in my relationship with Jesus and was acquainted with its power to bring freedom. Consciously praising God in exasperating circumstances puts the focus on God's power over the ensuing enemy. In the story of Paul and Silas from Acts 16, we find Paul and Silas going about their missionary journeys. In Acts 16:16 KJV, scripture tells us that a certain damsel possessed with a spirit of divination met them: "And it came to pass, as we went to prayer, a certain damsel possessed with a spirit of divination met us, which brought her masters much gain by soothsaying."

The scripture goes on to describe how she continued to follow them around throughout the day, for many days, the scripture says, mocking them and crying out to them. Finally Paul got enough of this, and turned to the young woman, and commanded the spirit of divination to come out of her. This of course made the men who were making money on this slave girl's demonic power very angry, and they had Paul and Silas thrown in prison. The spirit of divination used here is literally interpreted as a spirit of Python according to Strong's Concordance #4436 Greek dictionary of the New Testament.

Pythons are quite the snakes. They do not kill their victims by a poisonous bite but by constricting them. The snakes slowly squeeze them until they cannot breathe, and they are left crushed beneath the power and weight of the snake. When the demonic spirit failed in its first attempt to spiritually imprison Paul and Silas, he did not give up but used circumstances to bring them before the magistrates and accuse them of being troublemakers; the result was a literal prison cell for Paul and Silas.

I'm sure the enemy was thinking that their spirits would surely be crushed, that the weight of the circumstances would silence them, and that the gospel message would be extinguished. But the enemy could not extinguish their praise stemming from their faith in who God was. And at the midnight hour they put their crazy praise on—the praise that makes no sense. Circumstances did not look opportunistic; however; certain circumstances call to us deeply, compelling us to look beyond our human eyes and see through eyes of faith, to look to the things unseen, to see the things that God already sees, and praise Him in spite of our situation.

As Paul and Silas sat in the direst of circumstances, imprisoned physically by the enemy, their faith pushed through. As they sang and praised God, their physical chains fell to the ground. The earth shook, and just like that they were free. The enemy had tried to choke them out, to squeeze them in such a way that they would be unable to speak. But praises are the antidote to the spirit of the python. God inhabits (dwells in) the praises of His people. God was in the prison, almighty, unconquerable God. And God was in my prison that day, the prison that the enemy was trying to put me in, the prison of hopelessness, despair, and fear. The facts of the doctor's interpretation of data told me I had cancer and that it did not look like a good situation. The voice of the enemy would say accept the report and make the best of your time. But in my heart, I knew better. God was bigger, and I would praise Him as such.

And at midnight Paul and Silas prayed and sang praises unto God and the prisoners heard them. And suddenly there was a great earthquake, so that the foundations of the prison were shaken; and immediately all the doors were opened and everyone's bands were loosed (Acts 16:25–26 KJV).

Later that day walking through the Aquarium of the Americas with Kurt and Zoe, I got a call from my mom on my cell phone. We were in the gift shop, and it was noisy and busy, so I stepped aside to try to hear her. She was excited to tell me about the Sunday morning service. She shared with me several accounts of what was happening on my behalf,

> And if the Spirit of Him who raised Jesus from the dead lives in you, He who raised Christ Jesus from the dead will also give life to your mortal bodies through His Spirit, who lives in you (Romans 8:11 AMP).

testimonies of the prayers going up and individuals who were standing with her and believing for us.

I would like to make clear she was not saying they were sending good thoughts or positive energy my way. I would hear this phrase from time to time from well-meaning individuals who clearly had no idea how to reach outside of human soul energy and plug into the power of the Living God. There is no real powerful energy supply that we generate from within ourselves or of ourselves that has power to heal, deliver, or set free the captive. Life-changing power, life-giving power comes from the lifegiver Jesus Christ, and aside from Him, on our own, we fall flat. You can plug in, but there will be no supernatural power.

What stood out to me the most from my phone conversation with my mom was how the children's Sunday school class had made me a poster. She described the poster to me over the phone.

"Gina, the children made you a poster from the story of David and Goliath. They've drawn a picture in crayon with the words, 'The God in you is bigger than the giant before you' in big letters across the top of the construction paper."

I was blown away. Right there in the Aquarium of the Americas on a Sunny afternoon in late August God was confirming His Word to me. It was not a coincidence I had taught that lesson the week before. It was not by happenstance that I had been encouraging myself from this children's lesson. Out of the mouth of babes God was reminding me, reminding me of who He was, the God of impossible situations. I am thankful; I am breathing in His presence. I love that He can be anywhere, anytime. My faith was receiving a supplement. We take supplements to support our immune systems and help maintain our health. For me this Word from God through these little children was a dose of much-needed supplement giving me strength for the day, strength to believe.

The next day we realized that we would not make it on to Florida. We would have to cut the trip short because my doctor had called and my tests were scheduled for later that week. We spent the last day touring the beautiful Oak Alley Plantation on the Mighty Mississippi.

I was now beginning to take in each moment—the beauty of the oaks the grandeur of the river…life! But I was still struggling. With each beautiful moment came an afterthought: would this be the last time? I hated these thoughts. I wanted to have the faith of David to run head on in the face of my giants with only five stones and slingshot, dressed not in my own armor but in the armor of God.

But fear, like a dubious feign, kept lurking around to pounce on me. In the midst of my rising faith was a question tormenting me. In the back of my mind I was thinking, what if God wants me dead? This was a question I did not like and did not want to address.

This is hard to write, but I don't think I'm the only person who's had these thoughts. Who has not had questions about the motives and will of God? I was just beginning to walk out this valley of the shadow of death, and each day God would bring me closer to His divine loving character and His unchanging truth.

On the return trip home, I experienced excruciating pain again. We stopped to spend the night in Monroe, Louisiana, a halfway point, and I was miserable. I was praying, Kurt was praying, and I'm sure others were also, but I found myself up most of the night, unable to find a comfortable place. I was pacing the floors, and each uncomfortable physical pain was accompanied by a spiritual attack in my mind—mainly fear, the what-if fear. What if my liver fails?

Morning came, and the pain was subsiding. This quick vacation began with the thought of running away from it all, but there would be no running away. I would have to go back and face this giant and fight with the tools my God would give me. Some tools I already possessed, others I had forgotten how to use, and still more I would discover for the first time.

Chapter 4
FAITH CHALLENGED
(GETTING A GOOD LOOK AT THE ENEMY)

The first thing we did when we got home, after unpacking, of course, was to call on the elders of the church. I would be going for more tests, and one was to look in my lower abdomen, which had not been done previously. The other was the colonoscopy. We were intent on following what the scripture would outline for us to do. The doctors were going to outline their thoughts and prepare a process, so we needed, on the spiritual side, to do our due diligence. Calling on the church and having them anoint me with oil was a must in first steps. James 5:14 KJV says this: "Is any sick among you? Let him call for the elders of the church, and let them pray over him, anointing him with oil in the name of the Lord."

The tests came, and the news was that there was nothing else on the CT scan except what they had seen before. The colonoscopy showed only one tumor in my lower colon. He let us know that he tattooed it in order for it to be removed for surgery. My kids were pretty excited that Mom had gotten a tattoo. I was glad I could give them some humor. So one tumor in the colon—that was good in the scope of what all was going on. Yes, that was good news! Praise God. So now we would meet with the oncologist.

I will never forget that first trip to the oncologist. I think even today I have some PTSD from this first visit with him. I would learn that by nature oncologists are not geared to be the most positive of fellows. The very nature of their calling/profession is one where they routinely see suffering and death and are the bearers of much bad news. So positivity is not something they exude. I only say this not because I have extensive knowledge with various oncologists, but I have experience with mine and have discussed his personality with nurses and surgeons acquainted with the field; it does seem to be a thing. It's my observation that you shouldn't go in expecting them to give you the news and then break out into a rendition of "Somewhere over the Rainbow" or "Tomorrow" from *Annie*. Hope is a precious thing and something I was not about to receive much of in the next half hour that I would be meeting with him.

"Hope" is the thing with feathers—

That perches in the soul—

And sings the tune without the words—

And never stops—at all.

Emily Dickinson

My oncologist came into the examining room, his demeanor solemn and his brow furrowed. Kurt and I sat there waiting to hear what he would say. I really did not know anything more than what I had learned from the previous doctors. I had purposefully not run to the Internet and Googled for more information. I did not need more bad news or news that would be inaccurate, so I had not allowed myself to perform the proverbial Google.

He had my paper work in his hand. He introduced himself to Kurt and me, sat down on his rolling chair, and rolled right up in front of me.

He began, "So, Mrs. Routon, you have cancer. Would you like to know about your cancer? Because some people do not."

I could not imagine not wanting to know. Yes, I wanted to know. Then it came.

"Well, Mrs. Routon," he said looking at my paper work, "I see here you have cancer in your colon, your liver, and your lung."

"What?" Kurt and I were both saying simultaneously out loud, rather anxiously. "Lung?"

I had not heard that before. "What do you mean, in my lung?"

We were alarmed, and it was showing. He quickly backtracked. Actually he rolled back from us in his rolling chair.

"Well, it is only very small, like the end of a pen." He pointed to the end of his pen. "And we don't even know if it is cancer. It is too small to biopsy. It's just something we will watch and check in a year."

My mind was screaming, "Then why did you say it so matter-of-factly that it was cancer when you don't even know? Hello? There is enough bad news here today. Let's keep it on target and accurate."

Then he explained that the tumor from my colon had gone from my colon to my liver, and this was what was causing the pain.

"We call this colorectal liver metastasis disease."

And there it was—an official name for my diagnosis.

He continued, "What that means is that the cancer has left its point of origin and, in your case, has traveled to your liver."

He then explained the different stages of the disease, stage I, stage II, and stage III. "But you, Mrs. Routon, have stage IV."

My mind was whirling again. Stage IV?

Well, I'm telling you that I was not doing well on the inside at this point. I did not know a lot about cancer, but I knew enough to know that *metastasized* and *stage IV* in the same sentence were not good words. He went on to explain that surgery, in my case, would not be an option. He would make me an appointment with a surgeon so that we could discuss possibilities, but he was not hopeful for this. Because of the size and location of the tumors, surgery would require them to remove too much of my liver for it to remain viable. He explained again that I had five tumors in my liver, and one was quite large, measuring 9.7 by 8 centimeters, roughly the size of a baseball. My only option at this time, quite frankly, would be chemotherapy. He again stressed that it was my only option. He said that we would just have to wait and see what happened.

In my mind questions were circling like buzzards on a hot Texas plain. Chemo? No surgery? Stage IV? How could this be real? It felt like a bad dream.

He explained the chemotherapy treatment would be ongoing for six months (twelve doses of chemotherapy), administered every two weeks for six months. In the meantime I would continue to get CT scans to monitor my progress. He went on to say that I would never be cancer free. These words hit me like a hammer. I was not liking the *never* word. He said that in the past, before this chemo treatment was available, people in my condition lived three to six months, but now with chemo they were able to extend that time. Again in my case we would just have to wait and see how I responded to the chemo.

I wanted to hear some words of hope, so I said in my despair, "Can't I have a liver transplant?"

Oh, no, I would be on transplant meds the rest of my life—that was not an option. He did, however, say that there were always miracles and that he believed in miracles. So I promptly asked him if he had ever seen a miracle in a case like mine.

"No...no," he said with his furrowed brow and shaking his head side to side.

Then why did he even tell me he believed? He had basically just said to me, in my words, "Lady, you are dying, and the only hope for you is a miracle." That was what I heard.

He explained that the surgeon he would send me to early in the next week would insert a port. A port is a small flexible tube inserted in a large vein near your heart. He explained it would be better to administer the chemo through this port; it would be better for me and better for my veins. I think he said something about making an appointment, but I just could not hear anymore.

I left his office and fled to the car. I was becoming undone and unhinged and not in a good way. Sitting in the passenger's side of the car, I started crying, not soft weeping tears but uncontrollable and loud. I don't really remember exactly what I was saying, but it was something about not wanting to die. I thought I would lose my mind. I could not process this information.

Up until now I had been holding out for some good news—some hope. I thought although it was cancer, it would be simple, manageable, treatable, and easy to take care of. I had been looking for the bright side of this thing, but apparently, from this report, there was not a bright side. The words were unbearable. Kurt had to pull the car over quickly to try to calm my hysteria. Fortunately the park was nearby, so he pulled in. Reaching over to the passenger side, he held me close and tried to comfort me.

I had to call my mom; I had to tell her. Kurt asked me if I would rather he do it, and I said no, that I would do it. My cries were not better as I talked to my mom on the cell phone. I told her it was stage IV and that I would have to have chemo; surgery was not an option at this time. I told her I thought I would lose my mind and that I didn't think I could take this news. She said she was on her way. She and Dad were on their way. I needed my family, and they needed to see me. My dad would often say from this point on, "I need to look at you in your eyes to see that you're OK."

The doctor's office had been beeping in on my cell phone call with my mom, so I said good-bye to her and called them back. Apparently in my haste to leave the office I did not stop by the check-out desk.

The nurse at the other end of the line said, "Mrs. Routon, we've made an appointment for you to meet with the surgeon to have your port inserted."

I said something about wanting a second opinion. I was frantic. I was in denial, and this was happening way too fast. Somebody needed to slow it down, and I meant it.

Then the nurse said, "Well, Mrs. Routon, if you're going to get a second opinion, you better get it quick because you have cancer, and it is stage IV."

OK, well, if I didn't get it from the oncologist, his nurse was going to make sure I understood. We did not have a lot of time to mess around here; we needed to get on it. This reinforced the thought that death might be imminent.

I called my mom back and told her just to wait until the weekend was over and to come the next week when I would be having the procedure for the port. It was probably best for us all so that we would have time to process and pull ourselves together. I chose at this time not to tell anyone, including my children, about the mention of cancer in my lung. After all it was not confirmed. I did, however, tell my mom.

She said, "Don't you worry about it. I know people who have had anomalies in their lung that are not anything to worry about."

Kurt and I were agreeing with her. We would not accept a "well, it could be" diagnosis in my lung. We gave it to God. We had plenty of confirmed concerns before us to pray for.

I guess you could ask, "Well, what happened to your faith?"

It was being assaulted. The enemy was challenging me.

Kurt, in an effort to encourage and remind me of the Lord's Word to me, would ask, "What did the Lord say to you, Gina? Remember His Word to you that night in the hospital."

"Be not afraid," I said, but it was so hard.

The enemy was roaring loudly. Whose report would I believe? I knew who I belonged to; I knew who had faithfully been mine. I knew Him. He had never failed me, never forsaken me, and never left me alone. He was with me now, my precious Jesus, my victor, my redeemer, my healer. I would need to grasp and hold tightly to Him. And when I was unable, He always had a firm grip on me; nothing could pluck me from His hand. And nothing had taken Him by surprise on this day.

I went back home and went to the Word, the Word of God, the Word that superseded every other word, the truth, God's truth. I needed to read His report.

I opened up the Word of God to settle a question. What if He wanted me dead? What if I was done? This was not the first time I had asked myself this question. Early in my Christian walk, when I was about nineteen I had been seeking a closer walk with the Lord, asking Him to baptize me in His Holy Spirit. Kneeling down beside my living room couch, I heard Him whisper the words, "Do you trust me?"

At that time I was preparing for a small surgical procedure that would require that I be put to sleep and was apprehensive about it. That night as I prayed, I answered the Lord with a resounding yes—I did trust Him.

"But don't let me die," I said.

"Do you trust me even in death?"

I struggled with that. What if I said yes? Worse yet, what if I said no? I remember surrendering to Him. I would describe it in one word, freedom, or as country music star Carrie Underwood would sing in the song she made famous, "Jesus take the wheel." I was letting God take control and trusting Him with everything.

That's a funny analogy in the seriousness of this question, but quite literally God wants us to trust Him unconditionally no matter what the circumstance. We can look at Job and his words: "Though he slay me, yet will I trust in him." Job 13:15 The trust extends even unto death.

As I spoke that sweet and fully surrendered yes to Jesus that evening, I was baptized in the Holy Spirit and began to speak in an Acts 2 prayer language. He had access to my deepest fear.

Isn't that what He wants, access to every part of us? He wants us laying down self, giving up our own ideas and plans, and living for Him. He is not afraid of our questions. His love is unconditional, and He wants the very best for us always. I respect the right that God is sovereign, and His judgments are righteous. Even in death how sweet it is for the saints of God: "Though he slay me, yet will I trust in him: but I will maintain mine own ways before him" (Job 13:15 KJV).

Now this question came back to me twenty-seven years later. But now it was more specific. Now I'd been diagnosed with this awful thing threating my life. Again, God would not be silent. He had first spoken to me that night in the ER out of His Word in Isaiah 37. So I was headed back to that chapter, reading it and absorbing His divine truths.

To capture the full story in chapter 37, you have to go back a chapter. The story begins in Isaiah 36:1 KJV: "Now it came to pass in the fourteenth year of King Hezekiah that Sennacherib King of Assyria came up against all the defensed cities of Judah, and took them."

I will summarize the story, but I encourage you to read it for yourself.

This king of Assyria, King Sennacherib, was quite full of himself and obviously quite a formidable foe because he had taken all the defensed cities of Judah. Now King Hezekiah was the next on his hit list, and King Sennacherib was not seeing him as a problem. He sent his servant Rabshakeh to Jerusalem to let King Hezekiah know that he was on his way. (I guess there was no need for a surprise ambush when you believed you had victory in the bag.) King Hezekiah sent three men out to meet Rabshakeh and to find out what he would say. These were his first words in Isaiah 36:4: "Say ye now to Hezekiah, Thus saith the great king, the king of Assyria what confidence is this wherein thou trust?"

Wow! Did you hear that? Does that not sound like the voice of the enemy proclaiming how great he is and then challenging the very foundation on which we place our trust? Then he proceeded to blaspheme the God of Israel and even went as far in Isaiah 36:10 to plant the question in their minds: "Don't you think that your God doesn't want me to destroy you?" (Isaiah 36:10). And then we hear his lie: "The Lord said unto me, Go up against this land and destroy it." He was using their own God against them, telling them that their God wanted them dead.

Let's get this clear. Satan is a liar and the father of all lies. He comes to steal, kill, and destroy (John 10:10). That is Satan's will for us, and he will lie to your mind and accuse and slander the character of God and even twist God's Word in the process to accomplish his evil plan.

In Isaiah 37 we see how when Hezekiah heard the news that he rent his clothes and covered himself with sackcloth and headed straight to the house of the Lord.

Isn't that where we should head when we hear bad news? It's not literally to the church house but to that private place with God where we know we can hear His voice.

Hezekiah had heard what the enemy king had to say, but now it was time to hear what the King of Kings would have to say. That's where we find Isaiah speaking to Hezekiah in Isaiah 37:6 not to be afraid of the words that he had heard where the servants of the king of Assyria had blasphemed God.

So here we have it, the conclusion of the matter. Just because the enemy shows up at your door one day and says he's there to destroy you—and, oh, by the way, it's the will of your God—that does not make it so. Remember he is a liar. Check those words with the character of God you see in scripture. Check it with the truth found in scripture.

I believe God was speaking to me clearly through His Word. He was saying, "Gina, don't let the enemy tell you a lie. I have come that you might have life and have it abundantly" (John 10:10). This was the truth of God's Word. His character is one of bringing life and restoration. Jeremiah 29:11 tells me He has good things for me and a future. In Psalm 91 His promise is to satisfy us with a long life. So I chose not to believe that nagging voice in the back of my head that said maybe God wanted me dead. Maybe it was His will. The character of God does not taunt us with words that would bring fear. Fear is of the devil. We must differentiate between the voice of the enemy and the voice of our Shepherd. And how do we do that? How do we come to know Him? His character? His will? We do it by reading His Word and spending time in prayer with Him. We engage in a real relationship with a very real God and Savior, a God who loves us unconditionally.

We must be mindful of our thoughts and not give the enemy satisfaction by meditating on his lies and henceforth throwing away our gift of peace.

1 Peter 1:13 KJV says: "Therefore gird up the loins of your mind, be sober, and rest your hope fully upon the grace that is to be brought to you at the revelation of Jesus Christ."

Chapter 5
FINDING SOLID GROUND

During the following days, I began to regain my composure and come to grips with what I had been told. I was finding my footing on the solid rock of God's truth.

Growing up on the black land of a Texas Polled Hereford

> He brought me up out of a horrible pit [of tumult and of destruction], out of the miry clay, And He set my feet upon a rock, steadying my footsteps and establishing my path (Psalm 40:2 AMP).

Farm, I knew a thing or two about sticky mud after a rain. Once I lost a brand-new tennis shoe in the black land muck. In Psalm 40 King David describes his plight by likening it to a horrible pit of miry clay. On that day, hearing the news from the oncologist, I felt as if I had been sinking into a pit of miry clay.

It was not the doctor's fault. I am reminded of the old adage not to "kill the messenger." I am thankful for the doctors and nurses who God allowed into my life. I am thankful for their gifting and care, for their passion to serve the sick, and for their expertise to properly diagnose, prepare a treatment plan, and give facts as they are presented. Sometimes that news can be bad and appear hopeless. Sometimes it is not what we want or expected to hear. But what we do with that information is our responsibility. And how we respond to the information we are given is a choice we have. Will we respond in fear or faith? Doctors are simply analyzing facts as confined by human reality, but when you serve the living God, you serve a God who works outside of the human condition. We must remind ourselves we serve a God of power and miracles who is not restrained by circumstances.

Again I had to choose which voice I would listen to and how I would respond. It was fear verses faith and hope verses hopelessness. And the response of hysteria was not working for me. It was definitely not a space I wanted to hang out in. The enemy was trying to damage my faith by assaulting my hope. Again through the prayers of many I was able to regain my footing.

I went home and pulled out the computer. I had not allowed myself to Google because I was protecting my faith and choosing carefully what I gave ear to. I had no time for false or negative reports.

Many things on the Internet are hearsay or conjecture. Some even reliable sites I found begin their dissertation on the illness with statistics and percentages on mortality. Hello? What good really is that information?

It was not good to me. I wanted facts of the disease and treatments, not what might happen or how long I would have to hang around to annoy my family. But amid all of that there were some solid informational sites.

My mom had told me she had heard somewhere that a liver resection was possible. I had not heard of this, and my oncologist had not mentioned it, so I Googled the information. In retrospect he probably did not mention it because there was not enough viable liver for resection because of the amount of cancer in my liver. I was, however, realizing that I did not have to sit back and take everything the doctor was telling me as an end-of-subject, one-way discussion. I would pray and ask God to direct me on this path and help me continue to find the right doctors and the path of healing that He would desire for me, all the while believing for His miracle.

In my online search I only looked at reputable establishments such as MD Anderson in Houston, Texas; Barnes Jewish in Saint Louis; and also Johns Hopkins University in Baltimore, Maryland. Johns Hopkins had a great informational video and even showed a video testimony from a woman who had a case that sounded very similar to mine. Only a few places in the country were doing radical liver resection surgeries where in cases like mine there was too much tumor taking up the liver to safely remove it. But I read in this article, and watched on this video, that they were doing an innovative surgery that involved a procedure to manipulate the liver into growing, increasing its size prior to the surgery so that you could safely remove the diseased portion and still have enough volume left for the liver to function. Liver tumors that were thought inoperable in the past were becoming operable with this procedure. Aha, they were offering hope. It is a beautiful thing, hope.

 In the article they described how the liver is unique in its ability to re-grow after part has been removed. In circumstances where the tumor is so large that it would be dangerous to remove they were using a new procedure called portal vein embolization. In this procedure a needle would be inserted through the skin and into the liver. The physician would identify the blood vessel leading to the side of the liver with the tumor and embolize(cut off) blood flow to that part of the liver therefore triggering the other side of the liver to grow. After a few weeks there would be enough healthy liver present to make removal of the diseased portion possible.

I shared this article with Kurt and my mom. This article was a glimmer of hope. We refused to accept that there was no hope. Jesus was our hope, and He would make a way where there seemed no way. We would chose to trust Him to make a way out of this "miry clay."

The following day I went to see the doctor assigned as my surgeon. I was gun-shy to say the least. What would I hear today? I was preparing myself for what I did not know. After all the oncologist had not given me hope for the possibility of surgery and instead gave me the impression that more or less he was sending me to this appointment to rule it out.

I guess the receptionist could see the look of apprehension on my face because after she checked me in she began to reassure me. "Everything is going to be OK. You're going to like him."

I managed to smile and say, "Thanks. I could use a different perspective."

My mom and dad had arrived earlier in the day. They had made the drive to be with me for the surgery later in the week to have the port inserted. They were waiting at my house while I went for this visit.

The doctor I was about to see was well known for his work in the field of colon/rectal and liver cancer. I did not know him, as it was not my practice to get to know doctors for the fun of it. I was meeting him today out of necessity.

So here Kurt and I sat for yet another doctor. When he opened the door, the first thing Kurt and I noticed was how big he was. He was as tall as the doorway and looked like a linebacker. (Kurt and I discussed this when he left the room; don't act like you've never talked about a doctor after he left the room.) The first words out of his mouth shocked me and made me laugh. Trust me, I needed a good icebreaker, and he knew how to give it.

"What the he**?" he said. "You're the best-looking cancer patient I've got!"

OK, the receptionist was right; I was liking this guy.

He explained to me the good news first. Apparently I was in really good health except, of course, for having this bad ass cancer—his words, not mine. He was very frank and had the art of using colorful language. He did not mince words.

I think somewhere along the way he had learned that one thing cancer patients face is what I call the wall of anticipation. You've had the tests, you're believing, you're fighting anxiousness, but still you wait, and waiting feels like a formidable wall—waiting for the news on the other side, waiting for the new paragraph in the story to start. And often it is the doctor who is holding that news.

I was so glad he did not make us wait, and I respected him for being mindful of the emotions that follow a cancer diagnosis. He did not keep us in suspense nor did he waste time with cheesy small talk. He walked in and got right to the heart of the visit. He explained why he believed and agreed that chemo was the best plan of action at this time for me. He described how he would be inserting the port and how it would look and feel. He told me that the chemo I would be receiving was tolerated well by most people.

He then followed that by saying, "It will knock you on you're a** for a few days afterward." Again he liked to use colorful language.

He told me that I would not lose all my hair as he motioned to his bald head. He said the first step would be to get the port inserted so that treatment could begin. The port would be inserted in my upper right chest and connected to a vein that leads to my heart. It would act as an access point for chemotherapy. Then what? We would wait and see.

He instructed me not to Google anything except for certain sites, or I could get wrong information. I told him I already knew this and was taking precautions. He gave me a list of sites to visit. He did not mention Johns Hopkins, so I mentioned it. I just said I had visited them online. He took a deep breath, wiped his chin, and looked very intent for a few seconds. I could see he was aware of what they were doing.

His response was, "Yes, they are doing some crazy stuff out there."

We did not discuss the procedure. I did not know at the time, but he knew a lot more about it than he was going to get into at this visit. He just told me that he believed the right step at this time was to begin chemotherapy and wait and see. He would monitor me with CT scans every three months.

I went home that day from this doctor with a renewed sense of hope that lined up closer to what I believed in my heart.

No man can tell you when you live or when you die. They have medical scenarios they can compare to and look at, but who really knows? In this doctor's words, he said, quite frankly, "You could walk out of here today, get into a car, and have an accident and die. I can't tell you how much time you have."

He went on to share with me what he had seen in his practice. Some people had big cancers, and some had little cancers, but size did not seem to matter. Some died with small cancers, and others lived with big cancers, so who really knows? Again I walked out not feeling so assaulted by hopeless words. The words did not give me false hope, but they did not give me impending death. They were simply...I don't know...we would have to wait and see.

But I knew in my heart the One who did know, the One I could hope in, and He would not disappoint. And although I wasn't privy to all of God's thoughts on this matter, I was going to contend for what I did know. God was not dead. He was very much alive. I was in His unchanging hand, and He loved me unconditionally. None of this was taking Him by surprise. He was in my yesterday, my today, and my tomorrow. I was going to have to learn to trust Him like never before. My faith was being challenged, and I would run, cling, and hold fast to His Word.

During this waiting time before chemo began and while the port was being inserted, Kurt, my advocate in this fight, called Johns Hopkins.

They are prepared to give you a second opinion. You can fly out for a visit or send them information. Kurt chose to call and spoke with someone. They were willing to see me for a formal second opinion. But with the number of tumors I had, they told him informally at that time their first step would be to give chemotherapy. The concept here would be to try to shrink the tumors. Kurt and I discussed it along with my mom. We prayed and felt at peace with the decision to go forward with the chemotherapy. Yes, my friends, it does take faith to let someone administer chemicals with mustard gas properties into your body.

The oncologist, my local surgeon, and Johns Hopkins all believed that this was the best plan of action for me. Also stage IV meant the cancer had gone to the lymph nodes. Chemo would go all over the body and attempt to slow down the progression. We would proceed with the chemo and would just have to wait and see what happened and discuss the possibility for more options later.

I went in early the next morning to have the port inserted. My mom, my dad, and Kurt were all with me. Afterward Mom asked the surgeon if he would do surgery on my liver, and his reply was that he was going to do something with my liver, he just didn't know what yet. Again we would wait and see.

Chapter 6
CONTENDING FOR THE FAITH

Beloved, while I was very diligent to write to you concerning
our common salvation, I found it necessary to write to you
exhorting you to contend earnestly for the faith which was
once for all delivered to the saints.
—Jude 1:3 NKJV

Wouldn't it be great if that measure of faith that was
distributed to each of us (see Romans 12:3) was never
challenged? I have likened this assault on my faith in previous
chapters as one who was fighting in the boxing ring. The
scripture uses various fighting words, such as wrestling,
contending, and enduring, words you would find in the
professional fighting world. I think if MMA (mixed martial
arts) fighting had been around during the Bible era, it would
have definitely been included in verse. We are not in a nice
fighting game with the devil. MMA fighting is not neat and
tidy. In my opinion it is quite brutal. Satan is not coming into
the ring just to toy with you. He is out to steal, kill, and
destroy (John 10:10). His agenda is to take you down any way
that he can. I'm reminded of a John Wayne movie where a
fair fight was defined as no biting, elbowing, or hitting below
the belt. The devil does not come in following a nice or fair
set of rules. He wants your faith! And he can be nasty in his
pursuit for it.

Yes, we have to fight for our faith! We are told in Jude 1:3
that we are to contend for the faith. The amplified version
describes it as to "fight strenuously." We are instructed in

Ephesians to be strong in the Lord and in the power of His might and to *wrestle* not against flesh and blood, but against principalities, against powers, against the rulers of the darkness of this world, and against spiritual wickedness in high places (see Ephesians 6:10–17). Why? Because we are in a *war*, and the ground the enemy is trying to gain is our faith.

As a Christian all that we believe in is built on our faith in Christ. He is the chief cornerstone. It is built on what He did when He went to the cross and rose again on the third day. Do you believe it? If you do, then that is faith. Faith is believing in something you have not seen with your eyes but that you have experienced in your heart. You believe having not seen. If Satan can have your faith, then you will be weak, defeated, and definitely no threat to him in the war.

Now I can hear some of you saying that Jesus already won the fight. He went to the cross, so we don't have to. And you would be exactly right. What we are fighting for is not our salvation, not our healing, not our breakthrough, not our deliverance, and not our freedom. Christ has already accomplished it all for us and said, "It is finished." What we fight for is our faith to *believe* that He did it all.

I think there are times that I would have in the past glibly said, "Well, of course I believe that," but then life happens. Maybe a son or daughter walks away from their relationship with God, a child you've trained in the house of the Lord. And the enemy mocks you in your mind, calling out every mistake you ever made as a parent. Or maybe a loved one passes away long before he or she should have. Maybe your finances are less than what you need to pay the bills that week. You believe, but the enemy is accusing you, hurling fear and doubt at your faith to weaken you and drain you of your strength.

But these are times when our faith is called upon to arise in the darkness, finding confidence not in our own selves or our own human strength but in all that Jesus has said and done on our behalf. Faith rises, calling us to stand up straight not cower in fear. We need the faith to walk through the fire, faith that will enable us to leap over a wall, faith to move a mountain.

Although I was careful to guard against listening to negative statistics, I was keenly aware that percentages of survival with a stage IV diagnosis were not good. I knew people who had passed from this disease and lives that had been cut short. I knew that odds were not stacked in my favor if I looked at favor from a natural perspective. But Kurt would remind me that their stories were not mine and that I must not compare my circumstance to anyone else's. I cannot answer questions of why some die and some do not, as human reasoning is limited and we cannot see all things as sovereign God does. Some things we will just not understand in this life, but we will understand it better by and by.

I began to declare this truth of protection from Psalm 91:7 NKJV: "A thousand may fall at your side and ten thousand at your right hand but it shall not come near you."

I was learning not only to read God's words, but to apply them to my situation by manner of declaration through faith and to open my mouth as scripture instructs in Matthew 21:21–22 KJV and *say* to my mountain, "Be thou removed": "Jesus answered and said unto them verily I say unto you, if ye have faith, and doubt not, ye shall not only do this which is done to the fig tree, but also if ye shall say unto this mountain, be thou removed and be thou cast into the sea; it shall be done. And all things, whatsoever ye shall ask in prayer, believing ye shall receive."

I had read this little motto somewhere along the way: "I believe, I receive." I took it and began to quote it, to say out loud His truth. I was conditioning myself, arming myself for the battle as a fighter conditions for a fight.

During the writing of this book, Rhonda Rousey is in the headlines as the undefeated UFC Women's bantamweight champion. Undefeated! Of her eleven victories, ten have come in the first round. And did I mention she was an Olympian, winning the bronze medal in judo in the 2008 Beijing Olympics? She has set herself apart as an athletic superstar, but this has not come just because of her outstanding talent. No, she has conditioned herself physically and mentally, disciplining herself and training for such a time as this. And we see these amazing results of her relentless will to win and athletic prowess. I'm impressed.

I saw her on *The Tonight Show Starring Jimmy Fallon*. Jimmy had heard that she liked to eat chicken wings after a fight. It was one of her favorite things. So he brought out this lovely plate of chicken wings—in the best way that you can make wings look lovely on a plate. I was astonished that she denied to eat them. I think Jimmy was a bit wowed by it also. She said sorry, but she was in training for the next fight. She would not allow herself to eat them.

I was thinking, "No way! It's a special occasion, for goodness sake. You're on *The Tonight Show*. Don't be rude, girl!"

But she was serious.

He asked her, "Are you serious?"

Yes, she was.

Now that is dedication. She knew what it would take to see the win. She was committed.

During the course of the battle I was facing, I became very aware that I would need to strengthen my resolve. I did not want to lie awake in fear at night or rocking back and forth on my knees beside my bed in the darkness, tears running down my face. Yes, I did both of these—the first because I was petrified and the latter because I was pressing through

---

So that the genuineness of your faith, which is much more precious than gold which is perishable, even though tested and purified by fire, may be found to result in [your] praise and glory and honor at the revelation of Jesus Christ (1 Peter 1:7 AMP).

---

the fear. I needed an arsenal like a fighter has in training. I needed to take in mega spiritual vitamin supplements. That meant reading the Word of God, listening to sound Bible teaching, reading faith-building materials (no crazy Google searches and no social media), and listening to praise and worship music and scripture on CD. I absolutely needed to be inundated with truth so that my faith could become stronger.

There were days—but mostly it was in the night hours—that I felt so weak mentally and physically there was pain. In those moments my dear Kurt would take the word, don his headlamp, and sit on the floor beside my bed reading the word out loud to me. He was my night watchman battling beside me, bringing my faith a much-needed lift and bringing peace to my situation: "So then Faith comes by hearing, and hearing by the word of God" (Romans 10:17 KJV).

My faith was taking some serious hits, and I needed endurance. I needed to strengthen my grip. Faith is precious. It was at the center of my hope: faith that God would keep me, faith that I would receive healing, faith to see my daughter become a woman and my two unborn grandchildren, and faith not to live in fear and dread. It was necessary to build myself up. I can't stress how important this was in my journey. The Bible tells us in Jude 1:20 KJV: "But Ye, beloved, building up yourselves on your most holy faith praying in the Holy Ghost."

As I read, listened, and prayed, centering my focus on Christ, my faith began to strengthen.

Fighters in the ring also have to learn to guard themselves. When you are learning to box, it is not just about delivering a blow to the opponent. It is also about endurance and guarding yourself against the damaging blows. Scripture also gives us instruction on this from Proverbs 4:23 AMP: "Watch over your heart with all diligence, for from it flow the springs of life."

The enemy seeks out opportunity to sow fear and doubt into the life of a believer and to undermine faith. So with diligence we must guard our hearts. Keeping myself conditioned to receive from God came down to guarding the gates into my life. What was I giving my eyes to watching, my ears to hearing, and my mouth to speaking? Did they pertain to life or death?

I would learn to contend for this faith. One thing a contender headed for the ring needs is a good fight song to encourage him or her for the ensuing battle. My fight song heading into chemo was a song from Hosanna Integrity music. When this music first came out in the eighties, it was controversial for some in the church because it was unlike traditional church music. But I love that many of the songs were scriptures set to music. By singing these songs, the Word was being sown into my heart. The song I chose as my fight song was "Mighty Warrior" by Randy Rothwell. I sang these words as a declaration of truth over my situation. The theme was one that addressed Jesus as our commander in Chief, the one who has all authority. He is the one who leads us and gives us victory over the enemy. It talks about our habitation being fashioned for the Lords presence and that he has all authority. It further declares that Satan has no authority.

I would sing this song in my bedroom before chemo treatments, stomping around in my room with my fist raised. Scripture tells us that as Christians our bodies are temples of the Holy Spirit. So I could envision myself, my body, belonging to Christ. I was not my own. I was His, bought with the price of God's own Son. 1 Corinthians 6:20 KJV says: "For ye are bought with a price therefore glorify God in your body, and in your spirit, which are God's."

Satan had no say so about what would happen to my body. I belonged to God. Ownership of my body I entrusted to God. Therefore He had final say about what happened to this body. Disease would have no authority in my body because Christ had given us authority over sickness (Matthew 10:1). I may have looked silly marching around singing my song, declaring His truth, but I didn't care. I was doing what I had to do to strengthen my faith.

I am forever thankful to those who were contending with me. People from Zoe's Christian school, people I barely knew, gave me faith-based CDs to listen to and books to read through the day. I had devotions for the morning and devotions for the evening.

One dear friend sent me an MP3 music download of the character/attributes of God from Genesis to Revelation. Many times I chose to listen to it at night lying in bed with my earbuds or during chemo treatments. It was a reminder of who He was. I listened to the same worship CD practically every night to fall asleep. Kurt and I can probably sing every song from the Passion Band's 2002 CD, *Our Love Is Loud*. I know there were nights he was probably sick of hearing it, but he did not complain. And amazingly it worked liked an anti-anxiety pill for me and kept my focus on the one who was bigger than all my fears.

Thank God I was not in this alone. Thank God for the body of believers surrounding me and for the great cloud of witnesses who went before us. I am including an insert following this chapter from Hebrews 11, so aptly entitled

The Roll Call of Faith. I encourage you to read it and not skip over. It will build your faith and strengthen your resolve whatever position on your journey.

THE ROLL CALL OF FAITH
HEBREWS 11
KJV

Now faith is the substance of things hoped for, the evidence of things not seen.

² For by it the elders obtained a good report.

³ Through faith we understand that the worlds were framed by the word of God, so that things which are seen were not made of things which do appear.

⁴ By faith Abel offered unto God a more excellent sacrifice than Cain, by which he obtained witness that he was righteous, God testifying of his gifts: and by it he being dead yet speaketh.

⁵ By faith Enoch was translated that he should not see death; and was not found, because God had translated him: for before his translation he had this testimony, that he pleased God.

⁶ But without faith it is impossible to please him: for he that cometh to God must believe that he is, and that he is a rewarder of them that diligently seek him.

⁷ By faith Noah, being warned of God of things not seen as yet, moved with fear, prepared an ark to the saving of his house; by the which he condemned the world, and became heir of the righteousness which is by faith.

[8] By faith Abraham, when he was called to go out into a place which he should after receive for an inheritance, obeyed; and he went out, not knowing whither he went.

[9] By faith he sojourned in the land of promise, as in a strange country, dwelling in tabernacles with Isaac and Jacob, the heirs with him of the same promise:

[10] For he looked for a city which hath foundations, whose builder and maker is God.

[11] Through faith also Sara herself received strength to conceive seed, and was delivered of a child when she was past age, because she judged him faithful who had promised.

[12] Therefore sprang there even of one, and him as good as dead, so many as the stars of the sky in multitude, and as the sand which is by the sea shore innumerable.

[13] These all died in faith, not having received the promises, but having seen them afar off, and were persuaded of them, and embraced them, and confessed that they were strangers and pilgrims on the earth.

[14] For they that say such things declare plainly that they seek a country.

[15] And truly, if they had been mindful of that country from whence they came out, they might have had opportunity to have returned.

¹⁶ But now they desire a better country, that is, an heavenly: wherefore God is not ashamed to be called their God: for he hath prepared for them a city.

¹⁷ By faith Abraham, when he was tried, offered up Isaac: and he that had received the promises offered up his only begotten son,

¹⁸ Of whom it was said, That in Isaac shall thy seed be called:

¹⁹ Accounting that God was able to raise him up, even from the dead; from whence also he received him in a figure.

²⁰ By faith Isaac blessed Jacob and Esau concerning things to come.

²¹ By faith Jacob, when he was a dying, blessed both the sons of Joseph; and worshipped, leaning upon the top of his staff.

²² By faith Joseph, when he died, made mention of the departing of the children of Israel; and gave commandment concerning his bones.

²³ By faith Moses, when he was born, was hid three months of his parents, because they saw he was a proper child; and they were not afraid of the king's commandment.

²⁴ By faith Moses, when he was come to years, refused to be called the son of Pharaoh's daughter;

²⁵ Choosing rather to suffer affliction with the people of God, than to enjoy the pleasures of sin for a season;

²⁶ Esteeming the reproach of Christ greater riches than the treasures in Egypt: for he had respect unto the recompense of the reward.

²⁷ By faith he forsook Egypt, not fearing the wrath of the king: for he endured, as seeing him who is invisible.

²⁸ Through faith he kept the passover, and the sprinkling of blood, lest he that destroyed the firstborn should touch them.

²⁹ By faith they passed through the Red sea as by dry land: which the Egyptians assaying to do were drowned.

³⁰ By faith the walls of Jericho fell down, after they were compassed about seven days.

³¹ By faith the harlot Rahab perished not with them that believed not, when she had received the spies with peace.

³² And what shall I more say? for the time would fail me to tell of Gedeon, and of Barak, and of Samson, and of Jephthae; of David also, and Samuel, and of the prophets:

³³ Who through faith subdued kingdoms, wrought righteousness, obtained promises, stopped the mouths of lions.

³⁴ Quenched the violence of fire, escaped the edge of the sword, out of weakness were made strong, waxed valiant in fight, turned to flight the armies of the aliens.

[35] Women received their dead raised to life again: and others were tortured, not accepting deliverance; that they might obtain a better resurrection:

[36] And others had trial of cruel mockings and scourgings, yea, moreover of bonds and imprisonment:

[37] They were stoned, they were sawn asunder, were tempted, were slain with the sword: they wandered about in sheepskins and goatskins; being destitute, afflicted, tormented;

[38] (Of whom the world was not worthy:) they wandered in deserts, and in mountains, and in dens and caves of the earth.

[39] And these all, having obtained a good report through faith, received not the promise:

[40] God having provided some better thing for us, that they without us should not be made perfect.

Chapter 7
FACING THE FIRE

Chemo day had arrived. I was ready…well, as ready as I could be. I had been building my faith. I did not feel much fear. My port was in place. I was just ready to get it started and over with. I was sitting in my bedroom lacing up my running shoes. I had already sung my song for the fight when Caleb came in. He had driven to our house that morning and

---

He who dwells in the secret place of the Most High shall remain stable and fixed under the shadow of the Almighty [Whose power no foe can withstand] Psalm 91:1 AMPC.

---

arrived at my bedroom to pray for me.

Pray for me? When do your children start praying for you as a parent?

He laid down on the floor in front of me where I sat. He laid both his hands on my feet and began to pray. As a mom I was both proud of him and humbled by this experience. I felt guilty at the same time and so sorry because I felt as though I was putting my children through this horrible thing, and I didn't want them to have this burden. I was so taken back by this expression of love and faith, so thankful that as parents his dad and I must have done something right for him to know where to fall when the world got ugly. Falling before our King Jesus is a safe and powerful position. In this position we physically acknowledging that we stand not in

---

I will say of the Lord He is my refuge and my fortress:
my God; on Him I lean and rely, and in Him I
[confidently] trust (Psalm 91: 2 AMPC)!

---

our own strength but in the power of His might.

When I arrived at the doctor's office that Friday, they explained there had been a misunderstanding and that they thought I had canceled my appointment. Great! That was a sarcastic *great*. I was all ready for it, and now I would have to wait until Monday. This mix-up in scheduling turned out, however, to be a blessing. And this was why.

The chemotherapy treatment for me went like this. I went in, and they inserted the IV into my port and began the chemo. This process took four to five hours in office. Then they hooked me up to a portable bag of chemotherapy called 5FU. No joke—this was the name of it. I wore this home for forty-eight hours and returned to have it removed. So basically Monday through Wednesday I was receiving chemo infusion. How was having it on Monday a blessing? I would have my weekends chemo free! That was a blessing. So I went home that day to have my weekend and enjoy time with my family.

In preparation for receiving chemo, one of the things you will receive is an informational meeting with a chemo nurse and pharmacologist. You get lots of flyers and pamphlets, and I even got a notebook to organize all my reports and paper work. It's a whole deal I really did not want anything to do with. But, well, it was just what it was.

They tell you all of the scary things that can happen when you take chemo treatment. As if you aren't scared enough of the cancer diagnosis, now you sit down with the very somber demeanor of the person who gives you this news like the grim reaper. Now I don't know how you should act when you're giving someone this information. I've only been on the receiving end, so I will try not to be judgmental. And everyone is different, and we all hear information differently. I am first to admit that my perspective was probably a bit skewed by my adversity of having to walk this road.

The nurse who spoke with Kurt and me was very—I mean very—young. Like in her early twenties. She explained everything as if she was about to cry. She was feeling my pain? I didn't know, but I wished she could have just read off the information minus the emotion because I was not in a position to carry any extra emotion. Does this sound mean? I think it probably does. Sometimes when you have cancer and you're taking chemo, you might have days when you just throw kindness out the door. OK, there you have it. I'm not perfect and obviously still have a few things to work on.

The pharmacologist, on the other hand, walked into the room with his own handicap; I think by the way it manifested, it was a form of cerebral palsy. Receiving the information from him came with an air of "OK, here are the facts; now let's plow through it." It felt as though he shared the information from the heart of a soldier, someone who had experienced his own hardships with the realization that when faced with adversity you can't mentally go to the sad place, the place of looking at the wound and mourning excessively over the hand you have been dealt. A survivor gets up and does what has to be done on his day of proving.

So he gave me the information for a second time on the Monday I went in to actually start the chemo. He explained things such as it would make me extremely cold sensitive in my extremities. So I would not be able to eat or drink anything that was not room temperature, or I would experience spasms in my throat. I would not be able to touch anything cold, meaning I could not handle anything out of the fridge. At the time I had no idea that meant I would not be able to prep food for my family, which had been my joy as a mom and wife for thirty years. Exposure to cold meant the feeling of pins and needles in my fingers and hands. And if I exposed myself repeatedly, it could cause permanent nerve damage. This would also be true of my feet.

He told me my nails might fall off, and my hair could become considerably thinner. He told me about the importance of rinsing my mouth two to three times daily in a soda and salt wash because of the likelihood of developing painful mouth sores, as chemo would not differentiate between good and bad cells; its job was to kill the rapidly reproducing cells on its mission to kill the cancer cells. He explained about nausea and that they would be prescribing medication to help with that. I was given a hazmat bag to take home with me so if the line to the pump I would be wearing home were to come out, we would have what was necessary to clean up a toxic spill and a number to call for help.

He also said I could have an allergic reaction at any time. OK? But there was nothing the chemo could do that they could not reverse. The nurses stood by with antidotes. OK? None of this was OK, but, yes, I understood. I got the picture. It was bad stuff, and if there had been any other way, we would have been doing it. But this was the avenue set before us and apparently the one I was meant to take today.

So how do you mentally wrap your mind around sitting there in a chair for five hours while toxic medication is pumped into your veins and then loping on a cumbersome pump disguised as a purse that I would go home with and wear for the next forty-eight hours, even hanging it on my bedpost at night while the pump steadily released the chemo into my body as I slept?

Again the Word of God became my strength, my defense, and my truth. What did God say about what I was facing? I went to Daniel 3 and to the story of three children of God who when placed in slavery and forced to walk a journey not of their choosing stayed the course, meaning they did not submit to the will of a king who would try to force them to worship something other than their living God.

On the day of their proving, the king said (my paraphrase), "If you will not bow to the idol I have made, then I will throw you into a burning, fiery furnace." He even challenged God by asking them, "Who is the God who will deliver you?" I can't imagine what they felt, but I know what they professed.

(Daniel 3:16–18 KJV): "Shadrach, Meshach, and Abednego, answered and said to the King, 'O Nebuchadnezzar, we are not careful to answer thee in this matter. If it be so, our God whom we serve is able to deliver us from the burning fiery furnace, and he will deliver us out of thine hand, O king. But if not, be it known unto thee, O king, that we will not serve thy gods, nor worship the golden image which thou hast set up.'"

Now that sounds like some serious resolve, a proclamation of determination. Of course this infuriated the king, so he had them bound and asked that the fire be brought up seven times hotter. The heat so intense that the Bible tells us those men appointed to open the doors to the furnace and cast God's children in died of the intense blast of heat.

 Yet in the face of what looked like inescapable death, their faith did not waver. The outcome for them was in the hands of the only one and true God who held their life in His hands. Their trust was in Him, and because of their faith, they were thrown into the fire. But a funny thing happened that day—also because of their faith. When the king stood to see them incinerated, what he saw instead were not three men in the fire, but four! And the fourth was like the image of God. And not only were they not hurt, neither their clothes nor

---

"Look!" he answered, "I see four men loose, walking in the midst of the fire; and they are not hurt, and the form of the fourth is like the Son of God" (Daniel 3:25NKJV).

---

their flesh was consumed. They didn't even smell like smoke. King Nebuchadnezzar called to the children, except this time he did not call them only by the names he had given them. He called them "children of the Most High God." God had showed up to walk through the fire with them. God got the glory on that day.

When I read this truth, a truth I had heard since my youth in Sunday school, a deeper understanding came to me. I would be walking through the fire. I felt many emotions, but I would profess Him, my God, and His completely capable ability and willingness to walk through the fire with me. Yes, I would have liked for Him to rescue me before I ever had to have one day of chemo, but if I would be walking through it, I knew I would not be walking it alone. He said in His Word He would never leave me or forsake me: "Be strong and courageous, do not be afraid or tremble in dread before them, for it is the LORD your God who goes with you. He will not fail you or abandon you" (Deuteronomy 31:6 AMP).

I began to see myself in this situation as God saw me, not as powerless but as a child of the Most High God who by His power had made me an overcomer and because of His presence in the fire I would be preserved and kept unharmed. Although the doctors were there to administer, my God was in control. I was in His very capable hands.

I decided not to accept that I would have any nasty lasting effects from this chemo. I believed that God would walk with me through the uncertainties of my future with His complete certainty. I did not need to know how it would happen; I just needed to know the One in whom I trusted and completely rely on Him for the outcome.

So when asked how I was dealing with the chemo, I would just say, "I'm coming out of this *not* smelling like smoke."

Chapter 8
FAITH TO BREATHE DEEPLY

As the days went by, I continued to receive treatment and to daily immerse myself in the Word of God so that I could hear His truth and feed my faith. I cannot express enough the necessity of this action.

One particular book my mom gave me was *God's Creative Power for Healing* by Charles Capps. It is filled with scripture-based prayer for healing and health. Praying God's Word was my new norm. My mom would also pray these scriptures over me daily. Thank God for praying parents. I also had a daily devotional by Dottie Osteen that I read every evening. Dottie Osteen and her testimony of how God healed her of liver cancer back in the 1980s was also a tremendous encouragement to me. You can find her book *Healed of Cancer* at your local book store. I also listened to the Word on CD and preaching from faith-based Bible teachers on healing. Proverbs 4:20–22 tells us that God's Word is life and health to our flesh, so reading them was a daily dose of medicine for me. Reading and hearing them kept my faith in check and fear at bay.

I continued to have pain when I would take deep breaths. On the pain scale of one to ten, I was not experiencing that extreme ten, "Hey, guys, I feel like I'm being hit by a Taser," pain anymore. Why? I believe God just took care of it. But I had a deep, heavy pain in my liver when I would take a deep breath. I also had been unable to sneeze. The action of sneezing requires you to take in air before powerfully expelling an achoo. It was a nuisance and completely unsatisfying not to be able to sneeze or to yawn without the nagging discomfort but bearable pain. This also affected my singing. I sang backup vocals on our Sunday morning worship team, and taking in deep breaths caused discomfort. I don't know if it was my liver or the tumor in my liver, but it pressed on my diaphragm and made taking in deep breaths uncomfortable. I sang anyway. I refused to give the enemy any satisfaction.

I had become fixated on this idea of breath and what it means to have breath. Breathing is usually something we take for granted and do unconsciously, but because of this uncomfortable fullness in my liver, I was reminded of the tumor every time I took a deep breath , a reminder that I had been diagnosed with cancer.

I contemplated the very first breath physically given to mankind by God the Creator. I thought about Adam, the first man to receive this beautiful infilling of life in the garden, and how it must have felt to wake up to the face of God. I often felt as if God was trying to tell me something more concerning breath, but I was not getting it, and I knew it.

During this time there was also a lot of restless nights of sleep. I found it difficult to relax and uncomfortable to sleep with the chemo pump attached to me during chemo week. I did not want to yank the line out while I slept and have a toxic cleanup on my hands. On off weeks I recuperated and tried to live as normally as possible. But in the evening, I would lie in my bed in the dark, and peaceful sleep alluded me, replaced by mass random thinking. So what do you do?

Pray until you can't pray. Then what else? Well, I don't know about you, but sometimes I picked up the phone lying on the nightstand next to my bed.

One particularly difficult night I opened up Facebook and scrolled down. I saw a post by our state overseer's wife, Rhonda Brown. I love her Facebook posts. She is rather good at giving you just enough to make you want more. Many times she would post just short statements without a lot of explanation. I have not asked her, but I believe she does this on purpose to spark our hearts and minds and to entice the reader to think on his or her own. I might add that this is a sign of a good teacher, who makes you want to dive deeper into the subject matter on your own. Rhonda had become a great source of encouragement to me along the way, calling me often and praying with me on the phone. She, along with her husband, Bishop Tim Brown, made trips to be with me during CT scans and hospital trips. I was so thankful for this beautiful prayer sister and her husband.

So what was her post on Facebook? Have I made you wonder? It simply said "Ruach The breath of God" Immediately the words I saw reached out and grabbed me. Could these few short words on this post be the answer to what the spirit of God had been nudging me about in the past weeks? So on this evening lying awake in my bed at two in the morning, I thought I would just do a Hebrew word study on Ruach, which was not all that difficult with Google access on my handy cell phone.

During my late-night word search, I found the Hebrew for Christians website by John Jacobs. The website is a wealth of information and confirmation to me of what the voice of

God had been trying to speak to me previously. I will share what stood out to me here.

The very first scripture at the top of the page was from Job 33:4 KJV: "The Spirit of God has made me, the Breath of the almighty has given me Life."

As I read this scripture I felt the Word become alive in me. It struck me that there was a two-step process in play, the created physical body and then the very breath of God breathed into man to give him life. God had given me the life I possessed. My very breath belonged to God. He gave it to me. And it was creative breath! It was the source of my very life. In Genesis 1:2 when the spirit of God moved upon the waters, that spirit (defined in Hebrew as Ruach – breath or wind) brought a creative action. I was getting excited. Now I really couldn't sleep. The earth had been sitting in darkness, with out form, and void. The earth had been in a chaotic state until the breath(Ruach)of God came bringing a creative action.

I could picture God in the garden as He carefully and skillfully created Adam out of the dust of the ground and then breathed His almighty breath into Adam's nostrils, bringing life to the creation.

I have a book by Derek Prince titled *The Holy Spirit in You*. He describes in his book how the Holy Spirit brings supernatural life and health to our physical bodies. He references a scripture from Romans 8:11 KJV. I had read it many times in my daily reading; it was a scripture I was holding on to: "And if Christ is in you, the body is dead because of sin, but the spirit is life because of righteousness. But if the Spirit of him who raised Jesus from the dead dwells in you, he who raised Christ from the dead will also give life to your mortal bodies through his Spirit, who dwells in you."

The implication here as described by Prince in his book and what we can read for ourselves in this scripture is that when Christ comes in, our old nature, the sin nature, is terminated, and our spirits come alive with the life of God. Then in Romans 8:11 we see how the same person, the same power that raised the body of Jesus from the tomb, is living in the bodies of any yielded believer, and that power is not only for our spiritual bodies but for our mortal bodies as well. Prince goes on to say that the resurrection life in our mortal bodies can take care of all the physical needs of our bodies until the time that God separates spirit from the body and calls us home. After all He is the Creator of these bodies we live in. I will share here an excerpt from Prince's book that I find most enlightening to my situation:

> We must understand how our bodies were formed in the first place because it all relates together. Genesis 2:7 states,
>
> *And the Lord God formed man of the dust of the ground, and breathed into his nostrils the breath of life; and man became a living being. NKJV*
>
> What was it that produced man's physical body? It was the inbreathed Spirit of God that transformed a clay form into a living human being with all the miracles and marvels of a functioning human body. The Holy Spirit originally brought the Physical body into

being. Logically, it follows that He's the one
to sustain it. This is so logical, if only
Christians can see it. Divine healing and
divine health are logical in the light of
Scripture.

I suddenly felt and knew in my being what God was trying to tell me. He had created me; it was His breath that was giving me life. This was my scripture (Job 33:4), my word from God, given to me at this late-night hour when all was quiet around me. I could hear His voice loud and clear.

I began to declare this verse daily as I took precious breath into my lungs. It was His breath that had given me life, and I would breathe in its creative activity daily. I would believe that with each breath the Holy Spirit was bringing His creative breath of life to every fiber of my being.

I later shared this information with my friend Rhonda as she and Bishop Brown sat with Kurt and me for my first CT scan following three months of chemo. She listened attentively as I shared with excitement my new revelation, and then she added her insight.

She said that this made sense because "cancer cells are in a state of chaos; they are out of order not reacting as God created them." Her description excited me even more. I could picture His creative breath at work inside of me. As I began speaking the Word, God was bringing order to the chaotic state of my cells. His Ruach, breath, bringing creative activity as in Genesis 1:2, was at work in my body, bringing the cells into alignment with His design.

Death would have to flee. I became aware that this battle was not just about healing, but it was about life and death. I was not just encountering a sickness, but I was facing death. I believe they are different and that one does not always go with the other. In my case it was the threat of death being made to me along with the diagnosis. So I began not only to speak healing but also life.

The report of the Lord says in John 10:10 that the enemy comes to steal, kill, and destroy but also that God came that I might have life and have it abundantly. So His truth, God's truth, is what I grasped hold to. It was God's idea for me to have abundant life and the enemy's idea to steal that life and shorten my existence.

Psalm 91:4 talks about His truth being our shield and buckler. The truth of His Word was shielding me and holding me up. It also promises me in Psalm 91:10 long life. So as the enemy does, he would throw fiery darts at my mind to try to corrupt the truth of God with the practicality of the world's truth. Each time the enemy would throw a thought in my mind that was opposite of God's report, I would use God's Word, His truth, as my shield. I would often say my newfound verse from Job 33:4 The spirit of God has made me the breath of the Almighty has given me life to counteract the negative death threats of the enemy. This was something I had to train myself to do, to cast down every imagination that exalted itself against the knowledge of God and replace it with God's thought on the matter: "Casting down arguments and every high thing that exalts itself against the knowledge of God, bringing every thought into captivity to the obedience of Christ" (2 Corinthians 10:5 NKJV).

Faith calls us to step out of the realm of the way things practically appear and into the realm of the supernatural, calling those things that are not as though they are.

In Romans 4:17 we see how God changed Abram's name to Abraham, calling him the father of many nations before he ever was. God was calling him the father of many nations before he ever even had a child or the hope of having one. He was calling those things that weren't as though they were. It might feel strange at first, but this is how God instructs us in His Word.

We see Abraham's response in Romans 4:20–22 NKJV: "He did not waver at the promise of God through unbelief, but was strengthened in faith, giving glory to God, and being fully convinced that what he had promised He was also able to perform. And therefore it was accounted to him for righteousness."

Abraham's first step was believing what God had said. It seems that believing is directly connected to our confession. Abraham let God know that he believed he was able, and by professing his new name, "Abraham," which means father of many nations, he was confessing it any time he or anyone called his name, even when it had not visibly happened yet.

We also have further instruction on this matter in 2 Corinthians 4:13 NKJV: "And since we have the same spirit of faith, according to what is written, 'I believed and therefore I spoke, we also believe and therefore speak.'"

Here again we take those precious tenants of faith that we believe, and because we believe, we speak them.

In Mark 11:22–24 Jesus has something to say about how to strategically use the words of our mouth when encountering a mountain. He and the disciples had just come into Jerusalem and encountered a fig tree not producing fruit. Jesus cursed the tree. The very next day the disciples and Jesus came once more by the fig tree and found it withered. The disciples were amazed. So Jesus said to them: "Have faith in God. For assuredly, I say to you, whoever says to this mountain, 'Be removed and be cast into the sea,' and does not doubt in his heart, but believes that those things he says will be done, he will have whatever he says. Therefore I say to you, whatever things you ask when you pray, believe that you receive them, and you will have them."

The book *God's Prescription for Divine Health* by Gloria Copeland calls us to take notice of how many times the word *say* is used in conjunction with how many times the word *believed* is used. The two go together, one action following another. I have heard well-intentioned individuals pray for God to move their mountains, but in this example that Jesus gives us, He is clearly saying for us to open up our own mouths and speak to the mountain.

As children of God, we have been given the permission and authority to speak to the mountain that lies before us. By doing this we are expressing by demonstration that we trust Him for the impossible. But how many times do we stand there expecting Him to move the mountain in front of us when we have not followed the process He outlined for us to follow, to simply apply our faith to the mountain by confession of faith over the obstacle? He has already given us the go-ahead. We just need to know His will on the matter

(His Word), believe it, speak it, and receive by faith. Patiently expecting, counting God as Abraham did, fully able to do what He said He will do even when we haven't seen it but are fully expecting because Daddy God said so.

Chapter 9
CHANGING THE COURSE OF THE BATTLE

For You have armed me with strength for the battle;
You have subdued under me those who rose up against me.
—Psalm 18:39 NKJV

On the day after my first chemo treatment, Kurt was concerned about leaving me home alone, so Caleb, our youngest son, came to stay with me. His job as a crop adjuster offered him some flexibility, so he offered to come and hang out with Mom. I was mainly sleepy and felt as though I had no energy after that first treatment day and during that following forty-eight hours. I lay in the bed and napped while Caleb sat in the family room watching TV.

I remember lying in bed that morning somewhere between awake and asleep. I could hear someone praying in the spirit in their prayer language, and then I heard a phrase: "Today I have turned the course of the battle." If I wasn't completely awake before, I was now. It was so clear it was alarming, but not in a bad way.

I got out of bed, and my phone had a text message alert. It was a woman from our local congregation. She wanted me to know that she had been praying for me. I walked out of my room and down the hall to the family room where Caleb was, and I told him what I had just heard. We both praised God. I did not take these words lightly or brush them off as a half-asleep-induced chemo event. I believe I was hearing the result of prayers going up on my behalf. God was doing a work in me. He was healing me.

My prayer during chemo was that God would use it like an arrow, that it would only go to the places it was supposed to go and leave everything else alone. I was walking through the valley of the shadow of death, but God was by my side.

I imagine the valley of the shadow of death like this. A narrow path lies before me. Darkness like that of a dark forest at night is on either side. The path is lit but only where I am walking. God is with me; I am not alone. It is only Him, the One, the Almighty unconquerable one of Psalm 91, and me. I read this chapter every night before I close my eyes. Not only is it powerful as it goes forth to accomplish its truth, but it declares who God is and His position in my situation whatever it may be.

As I would go to chemo treatments, I tried always to have a faith-based book in hand or praise music on my earphones, or I would just read the Word. I could not allow my mind to sit there blank, waiting for the enemy to fill it with some vain imagination. I needed to meditate on the Word as it tells us to do in Psalms.

This is a different meditation than what takes place in Eastern religion, where one is taught to empty the mind of all thoughts. That is very dangerous. When you empty your mind, any thought can come and take residence in that empty place. As Christians we are instructed to meditate on the Word. As we meditate on God's truth, our minds are renewed. We are filled with right thinking and gain Godly wisdom and understanding. Depending on what scripture you are meditating on, you can find peace, comfort, joy, direction, and much more than I can list here. Everything we have need of can be found through the Word of God. As we mix the living, powerful Word with our faith and confess it with our mouth, then it becomes a two-edged sword able to accomplish the thing where it is sent. Consider this scripture from Hebrews 4:12 NKJV: "For the Word of God is living, powerful and sharper than any two-edged sword."

Then Isaiah 55:11 KJV says: "So shall my word be that goeth forth out of my mouth; it shall not return unto me void, but it shall accomplish that which I please, and it shall prosper in the thing whereto I sent it."

How does the Word return to God? It returns when we hear it and then speak it back infused with faith. And it shall not return void or empty. I began to open my mouth and speak His truths expecting His living Word to bring His creative process to fruition on my behalf, and I believe it to be true for anyone who will speak it according to Gods will in faith.

When the voice of everything dark would come around to whisper hopelessness, I would take God's truth and declare it. I would declare Psalm 91:4, holding it high, and I believe as I did that, the truth of God's Word became a shield and a buckler to protect me. The enemy is relentless, but remember he is a defeated foe. We are already overcomers through what Christ did for us on the cross. We must lay hold of that truth and believe nothing less. Reminding myself of these truths was necessary for me daily.

The struggle was real, and although I was learning to apply God's Word, it was a choice not to give into the fear, and during the evening particularly difficult. During these early days of chemo, I was often restless. I found it difficult to sit and watch a movie with my family. I could not relax. I would become overwhelmed just sitting there. Moments meant to be recreational would become anxious. Peace was allusive, and I couldn't seem to find it.

I remember one evening struggling, so I retreated to my bedroom and dropped to the floor. I was a mess, crying and in turmoil in my mind. As I sobbed my phone interrupted with a text message. I wiped my eyes and crawled across the room to look at it. To my surprise it was a message from a dear saint of God who we had pastored at another church. I had not heard from her in quite a while. She had battled cancer herself some forty years before, and God had been her victor, bringing healing and sustaining her through radiation treatments and surgery. Her message to me was a quote from Barbara Johnson, it said:

> Gina, you are a choice vessel of the Lord! His grace is sufficient for difficult days. We all go through pain and sorrow; but the presence of God, like a warm comforting blanket, can shield and protect us and allow the deep inner joy to surface, even in the most devastating circumstances.

As I was on the floor struggling to find peace, this dear saint sent me this timely message. I knew God was in the room, that He was reaching out to me through this dear woman of God.

But wait, God was not finished. My phone signaled yet again, and it was a fellow pastor's wife I had met briefly through another acquaintance some years before. Although I did not know her well, she had a beautiful spirit about her and was memorable because of it. I had to look at the name twice because I did not even know she knew of my diagnosis. But nevertheless, here she was, and obviously she had been hearing from God on my behalf. She had sent me a Facebook message with a link to a YouTube song. I was curious, so I clicked on it. The name of the song was "Cover Me" by Mark Condon. When I clicked to listen, the songwriter and singer, Mark Condon, began to give a testimony about how the song came to him. As he sang the words saturated my troubled spirit with sweet peace. Then in the middle of the song, he spoke, admonishing the worshipers, saying "Why don't you just pull the peace up over you like a warm blanket, over your minds." Not only was God giving me a message about peace in the very moment I needed it, but He was also using specific words—peace, like a warm blanket. I cried even harder. But this time it was because I was so humbled and honored that Jesus would show up for me like this and that in these evening hours, God was using these woman, whom I rarely spoke with, to reach out and comfort me. What if they had not been obedient? He was wrapping me up in a blanket. He was comforting me as a mother would pick up her crying, frightful little one and hold her close. I felt His love, and, yes, my fear subsided. I felt His peace. Everything was going to be all right.

I had many days of chemo ahead of me, and this was just the beginning. It seemed at first that six months was an awfully long time, but really it was going by quickly. With the holidays smack in the middle of all this, I found it to be both a blessing and also sobering. Life was becoming more precious than ever before. No longer did I desire to argue with my husband over some insignificant thing. Days with my children, eating a meal, taking a ride in the car to see the countryside…all these things became more meaningful.

I did not want to waste time. I wanted to do things that truly mattered, that were full of purpose. I became more compassionate, something I was short on prior to this diagnosis.

One afternoon I drove out to our local Marshalls to do some shopping. I was talking to God out loud in the car about seeing people and being compassionate and willing to be His hands in this world. No sooner than I had whispered this prayer, God put me to the test. There sitting on some steps on the sidewalk outside the shopping center was a woman who had fallen and was bleeding. I am not lying; it's the truth. Was God listening to me or what? I dared not look the other way. I walked right over and asked if she was all right and if I could help her. She explained that she had an eye disease and could not see well. She had not seen the concrete steps and had toppled down them. She had already called her husband, and he was coming to pick her up.

> Herein is love, not that we loved God, but that he loved us, and sent his Son to be the propitiation for our sins, Beloved, if God so loved us, we ought also to love one another (1 John 4:10 KJV).

Before I might have looked the other way and let someone else see to this woman, but not now. Things were changing in me. I was becoming less judgmental. Instead of losing my patience with the person who wasn't moving fast enough in front of me in line or the driver in the parking lot who was in my way, I began to consider what other people may be going through, what their day may have been like. Had they been sick? Was someone they loved hurting?

These are things I was less considerate of before, but now my heart and mind were seeing things from a different point of view. From where I was standing now—or maybe that should be from where I had fallen—I could see that none of us is immune to pain, hurt, or sickness. You never know what that person standing beside you in the grocery line may have been through that day. The same holds true for the person you work with every day or the person sitting in the pew next to you. As ambassadors of Christ, are we not called to be a reflection of Christ to those we encounter? We speak so much louder with love than we do with our preaching words.

I have been one of those Christians who believed I had words to straighten out a generation and put their feet on the road to righteousness. As a fourth-generation Pentecostal, I could pray loud, speak in my prayer language, preach, and teach the word. But I might pass a hurting person to make my way to the platform to speak that word or pray that prayer. Something is not right about that.

Without love we have nothing but empty words. And love is a demonstration. Love reaches out. I was learning to love deeper and purposefully. I was becoming more compassionate.

I do not write these words as if I have arrived at some place of perfection. I will be first to say I have not. I'm sure my family would confirm it, but I am by His grace moving in a direction with the intent of becoming more like Him, positioning myself so that when He speaks I hear. My prayer is to love more as Jesus loves, to see with His eyes, to be more understanding and less judgmental, less accusatory and more willing to listen before I speak. He has shown me mercy, love, comfort, and peace. Now I am compelled to give what I have been given.

Lord, help me, to not miss an opportunity to show Your great love.

Chapter 10

FAITH TO KEEP YOU

Who are kept by the power of God through faith for
salvation ready to be revealed in the last time.

—1 Peter 1:5 NKJV

Kept, phroureo; Strong's #5432; A military term picturing a
sentry standing guard as protection against the enemy. We are
in spiritual combat, but God's power and peace are our
sentinels and protectors. (Spirit-filled life Bible Word Wealth)

Summer was fading now, and the winds were turning colder.
It was fall, and I was approaching the midway mark with my
chemo treatments. I had accepted that it was God's will to
heal me, to give me long life. I had moved past asking God to
heal me and was now praising Him for my healing. I had
many discussions with my mom and Kurt about this subject.
We agreed that we had prayed according to the scripture and
believed for healing. We discussed that it just did not feel
right going back and asking Him over and over when we had
already asked and believed in faith. We felt that we needed to
start praising Him and expect to see. It was in His hands, and
we just needed to rest. There was no need to keep wringing
our hands and begging. We had petitioned our Father. I had
been anointed with oil according to scripture. I had several
different prayer cloths that precious people in the church had
prayed over and sent to me. I slept with one in my pillow case
and carried another with me. I was relying on His power.

When we read Isaiah 53:4–5 KJV, we see: "Surely He has borne our griefs and carried our sorrows, yet we esteemed Him stricken smitten by God, and afflicted. But He was wounded for our transgressions he was bruised for our iniquities the chastisement for our peace was upon Him and by his stripes we are healed."

Christ went to the cross not only to become the sacrifice for our sins but to take the stripes upon His back for our healing. Everything we needed for forgiveness of sin He did on the cross. Likewise everything we needed in our human frailties, including healing, He provided for and became our victorious overcomer. I can be victorious because He was.

I like the way Dutch Sheets says it in his book *Authority in Prayer*. He said Jesus did not suffer and die on the cross because He needed to beat the devil. After all He was the Son of God. He had nothing to prove on His behalf. All that the Son of God, Jesus, did on the cross was so that you and I can have victory through Him. Oh, what a great love our Savior has for us. Because of Christ, through His blood, I have the victory. I am an overcomer because He overcame. As our precious Savior was dying on the cross, He proclaimed, "It is finished." Three days later He rose from the dead, qualifying it all. He had overcome death, hell, and the grave. It was finished.

When people would ask how they could pray for me, I would ask them to pray that my faith would remain strong. Most folks want to pray for you, and I welcomed the prayers, but I wanted to be specific. I also had to learn how to answer when people asked me how I was feeling.

There are a couple of things we have to address here. Number one, I did not always feel great. And number two, I wanted to speak in faith. My answer became, "I am blessed and highly favored." These were true words. What good would it have done for me to sit and talk about pain, feeling tired, or any of the other unpleasant discomforts? No, I was not in denial. I was all too aware of my condition from the perspective of the human standard, but I was choosing to look forward in faith and profess in faith what I believed the report of the Lord was over my life.

Keep thy heart with all diligence; for out of it are the issues of life (Proverbs 4:23 KJV)

I'm reminded of a particular Olympic ice skater I saw interviewed during the Winter Olympics who had broken a toe during training. If you have ever broken a toe, you know how badly it can hurt. You can feel the pain from a broken toe all the way to the top of your head. It amazes me how something so small can cause so great a pain. Yet this skater skated flawlessly, and when asked later how he did it, he simply said he could not focus on that pain. He put it out of his mind and focused on the goal.

I wonder if David would have talked himself out of facing Goliath if he had sat around the campfire with the boys discussing how big Goliath was, how big his sword was, and how many causalities there had been at his hand. I think this could not be. I had to keep my focus on how big my God was and how perfectly trustworthy and incapable of failing He was and is. We serve a great big God! In light of His power, everything else pales in comparison. As I kept a close watch over my heart, my family did the same, for me and for themselves. They protected my faith on many occasions.

My oldest son, Aaron, was particularly intolerable to any down talk. Negativity was counterproductive. He simply would not have it. I know on occasion he encountered well-meaning people, church people even, who did not always share our same hope of healing. But he was quick to hold tight to his hope and keep the faith. On occasion when it called for intervention, he was, I'm happy to say, guilty of unapologetically correcting negatively directed speech with the good report of the word.

He has never been one to be afraid to voice his deep convictions, as all of my children carry the quality of stubbornness that prevents them from being easily persuaded. Aaron will and does passionately defend those things he holds dear. His wife, Lauren, shares his passion for truth and has a fervent spirit. She shared with me that when praying for me, she would use the word *annihilated* when referring to what God was doing to the cancerous tumors and cells. I really liked the ramifications of that word and would use it in my prayers also.

I too made sure if asked about my health to say that I had been "diagnosed with cancer," not that I had cancer. I didn't want to give any one the impression that I had taken possession of this disease and it had come to stay. My reality was that I was choosing to believe the report of the Lord, which was one of abundant life and healing. So my mouth

needed to confess what my heart was believing. Each day I
had a choice to believe or not to believe. I had chosen to
believe in God for healing.

To keep my heart and mouth confessing His truth, I
continued to keep the Word of God in front of me. I was
determined to keep the faith in spite of adversity. And my
faith was strengthening. I was feeling less anxious. There was

> Do not, therefore, fling away your fearless
> confidence, for it carries a great and glorious
> compensation of reward (Hebrews 10:35
> AMPCE).

a shift happening in my resolve. As I positioned myself daily
in line with God's truth, I would praise Him. It was strange at
first to praise and thank Him when as yet I didn't necessarily
feel it. My husband was getting used to the fact that almost
nightly I would get myself out of bed and do a praise dance
by the bed or kneel and thank God. I would pray for the
fruition of my healing and thank and praise Him in advance
for my healing or for whatever my need was for the day.

I had been reading *God's Prescription for Divine Health* by Gloria
Copeland, and she shared this scripture from Romans 4:20
AMP: "But he did not doubt or waver in unbelief concerning
the promise of God, but he grew strong and empowered by
faith, giving glory to God."

In this scripture she highlighted that Abraham's faith grew
strong and was empowered by faith as he gave God glory.
That is incentive to keep on praising.

It was becoming clear at this point that God was keeping me. So many of the side effects that you can have I was just not having, or if I did they were mild. If you did not know that I was having cancer treatments, you may not have guessed it looking at me. Again this had to be Jesus. He was sustaining me as I walked through the fire.

There were, however, occasions when I would feel sorry for myself. One morning after a cancer treatment from the day before, I woke up with the pump attached to my port and the sound of the chemo releasing into my body. The pump was hanging on my bedpost. It was my second day into the forty-eight-hour treatment. I was just disgusted with the whole thing. I was tired of it. I did not like the sound of the pump, and I did not like the smell.

I looked at the pump, looked at myself, yanked the covers back off of myself, and said, "Do you see this, God? Do you see what is happening to me?"

I was alone in the house that day, so I was doing a bit of wallowing in my predicament. But I got myself out of bed and went about my morning routine. I began with my morning declaration from Psalm 118:17, "I shall live and not die. I shall live and declare the works of the Lord." Then I walked down the hall to the family room, pump in tow, and found my spot in our recliner. I picked up my morning devotional my mother-in-law had given me right after my diagnosis. I had been reading it in the mornings. The name of the book was *Praying the Names of God* by Ann Spangler. As I opened it up this particular morning, the name of God that I would be studying and praying was Jehovah Roi…the God Who Sees. Imagine that. I was overwhelmed with His presence, there He was, right with me in my recliner as if to say, "Yes, baby girl, I see you, and you are not alone." I cried at how He honored me with His presence. I thanked Him for not being quiet but for answering me in my less-than-beautiful attitude. He loves us without reserve!

I was also continuing to get good reports from my blood work and CT scans. My oncologist watched my liver enzymes closely, specifically my white blood count and red blood cell count. They can take a nasty hit from the chemo. I also regularly had a complete blood panel. I had this blood work done every two weeks to monitor the effects of the chemo on my blood. The liver enzyme count had been high at my original diagnosis because of the tumors, but now they also had to watch it because the chemo was being processed through my liver. My liver was taking another hit in the name of the cure. But the name above all names, Jesus Christ, Jehovah Roi, was watching over my liver. And He would be the final say on what was happening. My liver enzymes were stable, and my white blood cells were continuing to remain in the normal range. My platelets also remained in an acceptable range. God was keeping my blood in spite of the chemo treatments.

The surgeon ordered the CT scans. I was glad of this because I liked the way he delivered the facts. I was able to go immediately to his office after the scan to get the initial results. No long wait—this was a good thing. He delivered the news in his usual straightforward fashion—not a lot of fluff or beating around the bush, just quick to the point.

He said, "I like what I see. The tumors are looking less vascular."

The next day I got the final radiology report from his nurse. She said, "It all appears stable."

I was unsure of what this meant, so I questioned her further on this point. She acted a little surprised and explained that it was a good thing. The tumors had not spread. It was just the same ones as before. So this was good news, and our family praised God. This had been the first CT scan since the chemo had begun. It was November, three months after my initial diagnosis. We took every opportunity to give Him glory for each triumph along the way. The glory would be His.

Chapter 11
FAITH TO RELY ON

Winter came, and it was cold in Missouri. The chemo treatments were ongoing, and God was continuing to sustain me. All of these chemo treatments were falling smack dab in the middle of the holidays. I found this to be a bittersweet

> Through it all my eyes are on you,
> and it is well, it is well with my soul.
> (from the song It is Well, by
> Kristene Dimarco)

distraction. I was discovering precious moments and cherishing each memory that we were making in a way I had taken for granted in the past and had failed to appreciate. As we decorated the tree, I carefully placed each ornament, and the thoughts of this possibly being the last time would taunt my mind. I fought not to succumb to these thoughts. My family must have sensed my struggle because Kurt and my children took every opportunity to remind me that I was indeed going to be around for lots more Christmases. But I think for all of us, as a family, it was heavy on our minds.

My precious Heavenly Father was also keenly aware of the heaviness of our hearts and the struggle we were facing. He did not remain silent. I love that He knows. He knows when to be silent, when to speak, when to sweep in and whisk us up in His arms, and when to allow us to test our wings, all along soaring beside us ready to rescue should we falter.

In this instance my help came by way of a star—how beautifully appropriate. If you are familiar with the Ozark Mountains, you know there are lots of rolling hills. Our home sits on one of those hills, and behind us to the east there is conservation land. We have a beautiful view off our back deck. He knew what it would mean to me, my Heavenly Father, so He gave me this view. It was a view of the rising sun each morning, and for this Christmas season, and for the heaviness of my heart, it was a star in the evening. I don't know the good people who put it up, and I'm sure they have no idea what it meant to a middle-aged woman with a cancer diagnosis, but it was everything: "And, lo, the star, which they saw in the east, went before them, till it came and stood over where the young child was, When they saw the star, they rejoiced with exceeding great joy" (Matthew 2:9–10).

So here it was, shining brightly every evening, carefully placed there by some unknown stranger, situated atop the side of a grain silo on a dairy farm just off to the northeast, probably a couple of miles from my home as the crow flies. Every evening it spoke to me to trust in Him, to let go of anxiety and heaviness and remember that God sent His Son for me because He loved me. It was a shining beacon of hope, pointing me, redirecting my eyes to the Son of God, my hope. And I could say, "It is well with my soul."

I continued to pick one foot up and put it down the next day, learning to have faith for the day and not the week. I was enjoying choosing gifts for my family, wrapping each one, and placing it under our tree in a lighthearted Grinch wrapping paper with goofy, fun bows. No, it was not very religious, but it was a story of the heart that spoke volumes. It is one of my favorite Christmas traditions to watch on DVD.

I had most of my shopping done a few days after Thanksgiving. This was definitely a first for me. I'm usually way too unorganized to have the forethought to complete a task of this magnitude early. But this year I had purposely tackled it before time so that I could enjoy the moments with family and not be put out with the rush. I wanted to savor each moment.

But of course there are always exceptions. One evening a couple of weeks before Christmas, Kurt needed to pick something up at the mall, and I wanted to get out of the house. I was on the second day of a forty-eight-hour chemo infusion, but I was feeling strong. He asked me if I was sure I felt like it, and I assured him that I did. He went out to warm up the car, as it was cold outside and as a result of the chemo drug, I was feeling the uncomfortable nuisance of cold sensitivity. I had on my heavy coat, gloves, scarf, and snow boots. And let's not forget I had the chemo pump in tow, slung over my right shoulder. I looked somewhat like the abominable snowman with a fanny pack. This was not a cute snow bunny look.

We parked the car and swiftly made our dash for the mall entrance, and just then the entire left side of my face began to spasm from the cold wind on my face. My left eye would not open; it was completely squeezed shut. Kurt was with me, and we just laughed at how funny it looked. It looked as if my face had frozen in a contorted winking motion. What else could we do but laugh? It finally relaxed once inside, but only after my face began to warm up.

We made our purchases, and Kurt strongly suggested that he get the car and drive to the door to pick me up. Now before you think badly of Kurt for not dropping me off at the door in the first place (avoiding the whole face-spasm episode), let me stress that he would have dropped me off at the door if I had let him. But sometimes I am stubborn and insist that I can do things on my own and that I don't need any help.

Did I mention that this was something else God was teaching me through my process of healing? I was learning how to rely on other people. I confess that this was hard for me. I have always been very independent. I do what I want to do and don't need anyone's help. Does that sound proud or prideful? Well, it should because it was. Somewhere along the way in my life, I had decided that I did not have to rely on anyone else. I was completely capable of doing it, whatever "it" was, on my own. I can hear some of you arguing here with me that there is nothing wrong with this trait and that it is a good thing. But I disagree. God himself is part of a trinity—Father, Son, and Holy Ghost, three in one. He gives us solid wisdom from His Word on the subject and the power of two or three. Here we see it: "Again, if two lie down together, then they have heat, but how can one be warm alone? And if one prevail against him, two shall withstand him; and a three strand cord is not quickly broken" (Ecclesiastes 4:11–12).

God said of His creation in Genesis 2:18: "And the LORD God said, 'It is not good that the man should be alone; I will make him a helper meet for him.'"

Have you ever worked where you felt you were doing your job plus everyone else's? Maybe this was in the workplace or on the home front. Wouldn't it be easier if there was someone to help shoulder the load, make the burden lighter? But to reap the benefits of having someone come alongside of you, you must allow them to do so in a manner or style that is all their own. It would require you releasing your need to have it done your way. Yes, they may make mistakes or get it wrong along the way, but we must be willing to accept this inevitable learning process, understanding that most likely we made mistakes early on also and that was how we learned. Accepting that others might or will most likely make mistakes is part of learning how to play nice with others. We are not perfect and can't expect that those around us are going to be. We need to learn to allow others and ourselves to make mistakes and give grace along the way. Then we too hopefully will reap grace when we mess up, and we do mess up most often due to our relentless pursuit of perfection wrapped in illusions of control.

I've heard my husband say many times that control is only an illusion. It is true if you consider that circumstances can change quickly and what you thought you had completely under your direction is ripped from your hand in a moment. In those times it's best not to be alone. Why? Because as much as we would like to believe that we don't need anyone or anything, that is false. While we all benefit from times of quiet meditation in seclusion, we were not created for a solitary existence. By insisting you go it alone, you are declaring your self-sufficiency, and that is dangerous.

God is our rock and is all we ultimately need in life, but He has given us people to walk alongside of us on our journeys if we open our eyes to see them, let down our guard, and allow them to come alongside us. We need not do it alone. How blessed we are to have the support of friends, family, and coworkers.

I was blessed with an incredible group of coworkers who stood beside me and took my share of the work during my chemo treatments. I worked fewer hours but continued to receive my pay. This was an unusual blessing. How fortunate I was that God had allowed me to work with this giving and loving group of people. If I had continued to insist in controlling every aspect of everything in my life, I would have been miserable and would have undoubtedly short-changed myself from the blessing that God was trying to give me.

God has promised to supply our every need. God chooses to use people. If you don't believe me on this, look at the examples given to us in the Bible. God used a widow woman with just a little oil and flour to feed a prophet. He used a prostitute to hide the men of God on her roof when the enemy was pursing them. He used Noah to build an ark that his family would take refuge in. He gave Saul a young armor bearer named David. And if people aren't willing, then He can use a raven as He did with Elijah to bring him food while in the desert. He can use a whale to swallow you and spit you back out if you're a Jonah and running from the voice of God in the wrong direction. God will make a way when we pray and accept the answer.

We could however miss the opportunity for our answer when it does not come wrapped in the package we were expecting. If you prayed for food, as Elijah did, would you accept the bread from a raven? Let's ask ourselves the question. Do we want God's answer? Will we choose to rely on Him, trust Him for His answer? Could it be that He humbles us by using the weaker things to reveal the weakness of what we thought was strong?

> But God has selected [for His purpose] the foolish things of the world to shame the wise [revealing their ignorance], and God has selected [for His purpose] the weak things of the world to shame the things which are strong [revealing their frailty] (1 Corinthians 1:27 AMP).

He may send relief in a way you did not imagine. God did not create us to bear our burdens alone. He will help you. He wants to help you. But we must choose to rely on Him to do so. That may mean laying down those things you thought were strong, even your own strong will. It might mean forgoing your version of right for His thinking that is far above ours.

I encounter so many people in the church and in the world who are filled with feelings of being overwhelmed with anxiety and stress. Not always, but many times this is associated with their need to carry the weight of everything on their shoulders. They are feeling out of control and are frantically grasping to regain the reins of a life that has become a runaway stagecoach from the scene of an Old West movie. I have been one of those people.

During my chemo treatments, I had no choice but to release control and accept help from God and from family and friends. It was not easy. I yelled at my mom one evening as she was helping prepare a meal for our family, a meal I was unable to help with. I yelled at her for laying the lettuce in the kitchen sink to rinse it. Everyone in the kitchen turned to look. I was horrified at the words coming out of my mouth. I was frustrated, frustrated because other people were in my kitchen, frustrated because I didn't feel good, and frustrated because I couldn't even rinse lettuce. My poor mom was so patient, as well as the rest of my beautiful family, just trying to help me. During this time I learned to release control and accept the help that God was sending me and become thankful. It was uncomfortable, but I can say that I have become a lot more relaxed. I found release from anxiety and stress by giving up my right to control the situation and trusting God with the outcome. Consider 1 Peter 5:7 KJV: "Casting all your care upon him; for he careth for you."

I was learning. With each day in the healing process, I was learning, learning to relinquish full control to my Heavenly Father, to trust in His unfailing love and accept with joy the help of the people He was putting in my path. I was learning to *see* and to *rely*.

Chapter 12

FAITH TO REST

For we who believe [that is, we who personally trust and confidently rely on God] enter that rest [so we have His inner peace now because we are confident in our salvation and assured of His power, just as He has said "As I swore [an oath] In my wrath, they shall not enter my rest," [this He said] although His works were completed from the foundation of the world [waiting for all who would believe] (Hebrews 4:3 AMP).

What does it mean to rest? There was a stirring inside of me, and this question continued to resound in my mind. I have mentioned that I enjoyed feeling independent. I also enjoyed doing. I am a high-tension person and usually have something going. I don't enjoy sitting and watching TV or even reading for very long at a time. I like to be up and about. I like to stay busy. This diagnosis was *not* fitting into my lifestyle.

Now it was everyone's consensus that I rest. "Rest…just rest," they would say—sit, relax, read a book. But sitting was not relaxing to me. Even going to the beach in the summertime would not be restful for me unless I could get up from my lounge chair from time to time and walk the shoreline.

Part of my enjoyment of the ocean is how it continually changes—the ebbing tide, the sand beneath my feet pulling against the water's edge. I love how it works in conjunction with the sunrise and sunset giving us art enthusiasts a new picture to soak in every day. It is always an adventure, not knowing what to expect but being surprised daily by the magnificent work of our Creator painting His picture in the sky. Stepping into the water's edge, I become a part of that picture, a portrait of His creation.

As much as I enjoy a good adventure, I did not choose this adventure I was on. I don't think I would call it an adventure even though it meets much of the criteria to call itself one.

Adventure is defined as an unusual and exciting, typically hazardous, experience or activity, especially the exploration of unknown territory. Yeah, it sounds pretty close, except not exciting in a good way. The cancer journey was not of my choosing and certainly not an adventure I was in control of. How could I find rest, rest internally and rest physically? They were connected, after all. Even though I felt my faith was growing and my trust increasing and that I was finding stability, rest was still a cloudy idea that I could not clearly picture.

I began earnestly to seek out God on this subject and ask Him to help my understanding.

Hebrews 4:1 has this to say about rest: "Let us therefore fear, lest, a promise being left us of entering into his rest, any of you should seem to come short of it."

As I reread this verse in context with the rest of the chapter, the meaning became clear. The Word of God is a simple message. We, however, in our humanity often make it difficult. What I learned was that when we personally trust and confidently rely on God, we find rest. Resting reveals our belief. When we are resting, we are not anxious. We find rest for our salvation, rest for our healing, and rest for whatever difficulties we may be facing in life that are turning our world upside down simply by relying on Him. So not only was I learning to rely on family, friends, and even strangers, I was learning to rely on God and trust Him in a way that I had not before. I was having a deeper revelation of His divine provision. I was to rest in the midst of trouble. This was a rest that did not come from the circumstances around me but from the spirit of God within me.

Hillsong United released a song in 2013 titled "Oceans (Where Feet May Fail)." I loved the song when it first came out, but after my cancer diagnosis, I found it hard to listen to. I did not like being "called out in oceans deep," but I was finding out His grace did abound in deepest waters even as fear surrounded me (as the songs describes). I was learning to keep my eyes above the waves, and my soul was finding rest in His embrace. What lovely words. I wrestled, and the words that I had found so lovely then now greatly discomfited me. It was not fun to go where my trust was without borders; however, my faith was indeed becoming stronger. It took me more than a year before I could listen to this song again. I had to find peace with it. Finding peace for me was accepting my circumstances in the light of my Savior's grace and drinking in His rest that He had for me. It was learning to float on the waters. Floating on the water is next to impossible if you cannot relax your body. It involves as much trust as it does technique. I was pouring the Word into myself. I was learning, understanding, and gaining knowledge, but it would mean nothing if I did not mix it with faith and rest in what my Father God's power would do when my power was useless. So I needed to just stop, stop wringing my hands, stop pleading, stop fighting the waves, and just lie back and rest.

Ephesians 6:13 tells us that when we have done all, just stand. So I stood and praised God with a big smile and determined will on my face and *not* with one of worry and anxiousness but with the faith that He was enough, that His grace was sufficient for me and I need not do anything more but to trust, rest, and rely on God: "For indeed we have had the good news [of salvation] preached to us, just as the Israelites also [when the good news of the Promised Land came to them]; but the message they heard did not benefit them, because it was not united with faith [in God] by those who heard" (Hebrews 4:2 AMP).

Chapter 13
FAITH FOR THE FINISH LINE

New Year's Eve came, and we praised God as a family that I was still around to ring in a new year. I was officially one month away from finishing my chemo treatments. I did not know what the plan was at the end, but I was taking each day and choosing to trust God with it. January is a time for new beginnings, and I was believing for just that.

Kurt's birthday was on the twenty-sixth of this month, and unfortunately my chemo treatment was scheduled on his birthday. I felt sad and guilty for him having to be in such a bleak place on his special day. However, he would tell me that there was no place else he would possibly be. Still I felt bad about what was not in my control. The reports from blood work monitoring the effects the chemo was having on my platelets, immune system, and liver count continued to remain in a good range.

As February approached I was looking forward to the signal of the last treatment but also feeling reserve because I did not really have a picture of what the future entailed. Many people were excited for me, but inside I pondered. Without the possibility of surgery, would this mean periodic ongoing treatments of chemo? As I understood this was to keep the cancer from advancing, a way to hold it back. This was not the route I wanted to take. I wanted to be done with it. My prayer was for complete annihilation of the cancer. It was what I hoped, prayed, and believed was done in Jesus's name. By His stripes *I was healed*; this was my profession. I was just waiting for the fruition. So I did not give voice to these ponderings. I also did not allow myself to let them become a heart issue. I had faith to exercise for each day, and that was all I needed. I did not need to allow myself to work out my tomorrow. God was holding my tomorrow, my future, in His hand, and I would continue to trust Him with it. I felt I was living in a crux between two worlds, the physical and the spiritual. What I believed did not make sense to the physical. It was not practical. My certainty for the future laid solely at the feet of my Savior.

I was due for another CT scan in the middle of February, and the final chemo treatment would be on the twenty-sixth, signaling just six months since this storm began. It felt like a lifetime and yet like a whirlwind. I was counting down the days to completion of the chemo.

Before the scan that month, I would give God praise for the good report I believed I would be receiving and then head to the surgeon's office for the results of the CT report. This would be my third time to see him, and I had still not heard any plan for my liver except that we would wait and see.

There had been no mention of surgery or even the suggestion that it would be possible.

The reason for this was because they honestly did not know. People respond to chemotherapy treatments differently, and there was a lingering possibility of liver failure because you just never knew how it was going to go (their opinion, not mine, I believed God was keeping my liver). So the doctors were functioning in the physical world, not my spiritual world. There had been occasions during the chemo treatments that I would have pain in my liver, and imaginings of what-ifs would pop in my head. My response to this was to lay my hand on my liver and praise God over it, praising God in faith regardless of the feeling.

The day came for the CT scan, and immediately afterward I headed for the surgeon's office for the news. As usual and thankfully, I did not have to wait for very long. He came in the room and declared that the report from the scan showed everything to look necrotic. I did not really have time to process what this word meant. He moved on to say that although the tumors did not shrink much, they were however indeed necrotic.

He moved to a white board hanging on his wall behind the examining table where I was sitting. I really had no idea what to expect. He drew a crude picture of my liver and then took a black marker and drew a line through his drawn picture, dividing off a two-thirds portion of my liver. He said he wanted this amount to be removed. What? I was shocked speechless and at the same time felt like a doorway had opened up at the end of a very long tunnel. We were going to do surgery? Was this for real? This was breakthrough news. We had moved from the wait-and-see perspective, a perspective that from all practical senses gave little hope of ever being free from this diagnosis. All along our hope and faith had been in the God of the impossible who we knew was able to step outside the scope of what the doctors could do to the realm of endless supply. And on this day we were rejoicing. Kurt and I were in an indescribable moment of emotions.

My surgeon went on to explain that he would not do the surgery himself or in Springfield. They did not have the resources to do this type of surgery. But he knew someone who could. He wanted to send me to Barnes Jewish Hospital in Saint Louis, where they would have the specialist and medical team that could make this happen. I ask him about MD Anderson because it is renowned for its cancer treatments and was in my home state of Texas. He said, in his very frank way, that I could go there if I wanted, but the person who wrote the book on the surgery was in Saint Louis. Well then, I should look no further. God knew full well in what state I would be living when this storm hit, and He already had the doctors lined up for me.

I closed my mouth to further discussion on the matter and said, "Saint Louis it is."

I would be seeing Dr. William Chapman for a consult. I asked him if this was to see if I was a candidate for surgery.

"No," he replied, looking up from his paper work to give me a pretty serious expression. "I'm sorry if I gave you that impression. This is not *if* you are going to have surgery. I'm saying you are going to have surgery."

I heard the words in my head and repeated them slowly to myself. "You are going to have surgery." Kurt and I were ecstatic.

He continued with more good news. He said he had looked at those spots in my lung, the ones the oncologist had mentioned some six months prior at my first oncology visit, the one we had not spoken to anyone about except my mom because there was not confirmation it was cancer. He said he had looked, and they just did not look like cancer to him. I sat for a moment, shocked that he had brought them up. I don't think we had ever even spoken of them at a visit with him prior. My CT scan, which is done every three months, always takes a look at my pelvis, abdomen, and chest. So they were on the "watch list," and I knew it.

He said, "You know, we will just keep watching them, but they just don't have the characteristics of cancer, and I do not think that is what they are." He had seen other people with similar things that were nothing.

I did not tell him that Kurt, my mom, and I had gone to God with what I called the what-if factor, had given it to God, and decidedly chosen not to worry about it. We believed this was just another something that the enemy wanted to use against our emotions. So like everything else, we prayed and left it up to God.

We left his office and couldn't wait to share our news of surgery with family and friends. The plan was to finish my last chemo treatment later that week and then promptly afterward travel to Saint Louis to meet the new team of doctors in my unfolding miracle. We were ready!

I wanted to ask him more questions, but he made it clear that I would need to get my answers from the surgeon in Saint Louis. I wanted to ask about the treatment I had read about at Johns Hopkins, but I did not. I was just relieved and praising God that surgery that previously seemed out of the equation was now not only a possibility but a target in my healing process. I left his office and headed for my oncologist visit. I was not dreading this appointment. I was somewhat giddy.

Waiting for the oncologist to come in, Kurt and I were still feeling the altitude of hope from the news we had just received from the surgeon. Our heads were spinning with the possibilities that lay ahead. At least now there were possibilities. The physical was lining up with what we had been believing in the spiritual.

My oncologist came in the room with my CT report in hand. I always got this news twice, once from the surgeon and secondly from the oncologist. They both worked together as a multidisciplinary team. He said that the CT scan showed that the tumors were all just dead tissue. So this was a visual for the word *necrotic* that my surgeon had used. For the first time since I had been visiting my solemn-faced oncologist, I liked the words that were coming out of his mouth—dead tissue. Praise God! He went on to say that they had shrunk only a small amount. He showed me with the measuring of his fingers how little. So for him he thought there would be no surgery because the tumors were taking up too much liver to remove safely.

But Kurt and I could not wait to tell him the news. We told him that there would indeed be a surgery. He hesitated and had a bit of a surprised look on his face. He inquired about the procedure, and we simply said we weren't sure how, but they would be sending me to Saint Louis to remove the diseased portion. I don't remember much more about that visit. We were just so elated. We were hearing words like *necrotic, dead tissue,* and *surgery.* All were good reports. I gave God the praise for making a way for me where there seemed no way. Kurt and I were smiling, and there was a sense of relief and excitement. We had been earnestly praying, praising, and believing even when the sky above looked dark and there seemed to be no break in the clouds. But today was visible proof of those prayers and the praise given in faith. A visible hole punctured the darkness, and light was streaming through. We were basking in His goodness.

Chapter 14
FAITH FOR THE PROCESS

I believe God heals in many ways. One is instantaneous. Some happen as we go along, or progressively. When we look at Luke 17:14 NKJV, we see this type of healing when Jesus healed the lepers: So when He saw them, He said to them, "Go, show yourselves to the priests." And so it was that as they went, they were cleansed.

As they went they were cleansed. I believe from the beginning God had been healing me. I was a miracle in motion.

There had been so many divinely appointed moments along this journey, moments where the presence of God became so tangible to me that I felt I could reach out and touch Him, and I did. I was the personal witness to His loving character and awesome power.

Even before my diagnosis, I believe God had been making preparations for me. Just two months before my diagnosis, my daughter-in-love Ashley had applied for and gotten a position at the Department of Social Services. We were all excited for her, as she had prayed for and desired this job. Little did we know at the time how important this would be for us in just two short months. As my diagnosis came, I had no insurance and no way to apply for personal insurance outside of the open enrollment date of the Affordable Care Act. I had no other choice but to apply through the Department of Social Services. Ashley navigated me through the laborious paper work and became my advocate. Unaffected by any obstacle, she was determined to accomplish what she put her hand to. I was able to get my paper work through the system in a timely fashion so that money and bills did not have to be something to worry over. Who knew? God knew. He was going before me and was with me.

As I arrived in Saint Louis to meet my team of doctors, I knew once again that God had gone before me. I also got the sense that everything was beginning to accelerate. OK, no feeling like it—definitely it was accelerating. Everything had geared up, and we were moving forward. The last six months had been about picking up one foot in front of the other and having faith and strength for each day. It wasn't that I was choosing to live in the moment; there was just no other way to live. I could picture myself as the children of Israel in the wilderness who had to depend upon God for their very existence led by a fire by night and a cloud by day. God would make daily provision by dropping bread to them. Literal manna from heaven fell from the sky each day. He was teaching them (and me) to depend upon Him and trust Him for every need. I felt like now I was beginning to see and hear the plan formulating, and God was the engineer. I had been walking out each day, hoping and standing by faith. Little by little I was seeing it come to fruition.

Joshua 6 tells us when the walls of Jericho fell, God's plan was that they walk around the walls every day for seven days without a word and then seven times on the seventh day with a loud shout at the end, and the walls would come crashing down. This was a plan for victory that depended upon a God-designed process. I was not going to get out of it. I was not taking the proverbial trip around the Monopoly board with fate attached to a roll of the dice. I believe that God had a plan and a purpose for my life, and I was walking it out and standing on His unbreakable promises.

One of those promises I kept running into. Three different people spoke to me on three different occasions from Philippians 1:6 AMP: "I am convinced and confident of this very thing, that He who has begun a good work in you will [continue to] perfect and complete it until the day of Christ Jesus [the time of His return]."

I clung to this Word, believing that God had indeed begun a work in my spiritual and physical body, and He would see to its completion.

As I walked through the doors of Barnes Jewish, it was overwhelmingly large. It is a teaching hospital. I did not walk in alone. Kurt was with me, but so was my Father God. I held on to Him and this promise and others from God's infallible

Word. I could see God's hand in guiding me to this hospital, this doctor, and this team of specialists. Even the fact that I was living in a state that could give me access to medical treatment at the forefront of liver cancer, I believe was guided by the hand of God.

The procedure I had read about from the Johns Hopkins website was about to become a reality for me here at Barnes Jewish. The liver specialist, Dr. William Chapman, explained to me about my cancer diagnosis and that it was not at all uncommon for this type of cancer to advance to the liver. He had seen it many times. He was factual in a hopeful way. He was laying out the process in front of me. I would need to go for an MRI that day before I returned home. He wanted to look at my liver and see how much he would have to work with. He thought I would need to have the portal vein embolization. He thought originally I would have to have three-fourths of my liver removed. The volume of the portion of liver left was very important. You have to have enough of the organ left for it to be viable. Therein lay the need for the embolization procedure. He explained that we would need to cause the good side of the liver to grow so that we would have enough working liver left after the surgery. Because of this I would need to have my colon surgery here at Barnes Jewish also.

The plan was to do the colon surgery first and at the same time perform the portal vein embolization, wait four weeks for my liver to increase in size, and then proceed with the surgery to remove the diseased portion. Sounded like a plan. But first things first. He scheduled an MRI for me, a visit with a colorectal surgeon who would work in conjunction with him, and a PET scan.

I left there feeling strong. It felt good to have a plan and to talk to someone who had seen this type of thing before. Thank God for men and women who choose to use their God-given talents to minster hands-on to people in need.

The next week I met with the colorectal surgeon, also at Barnes Jewish. He came in and was ready to do surgery.

He said to me, "We are going for the cure!"

I sure did like his outlook. He wanted to schedule surgery the next week, but I explained that I had only been off chemo for two weeks. I would need to wait forty-five days. Because chemo kills cells, it is necessary to be off of it for this recommended time frame so that the body will be able to regenerate and recover after surgery. We would wait forty-six. Clearly they wanted to move forward quickly to remove the dead cancerous tissue and affected lymph nodes. We left his office with surgery scheduled. The colon surgery and portal vein embolization would be done at the same time. Without this groundbreaking procedure, surgery in the past would have been otherwise impossible through human hands.

During this same week, I had a PET scan scheduled that Dr. Chapman had ordered. My surgeon in Springfield set it up, and I was praying. A PET scan is done so that they can see if there is any active cancer anywhere else in the body. I had not had one of these before and was unsure of what to expect.

The morning of the test I went in early. The nurse who took me back explained that this was a nuclear test. I had seen this nurse several times before in this imaging facility. She was of like faith and did not hold back in sharing encouragement. She would talk about God and the church. She was a help to my faith in the midst of heightened anxiety during these medical tests. She helped me keep my faith centered. I know God put her there. She helped me keep my focus on the eternal God of hope. I found these angelic nurses planted throughout my journey. They were another precious gift from God, a part of the provision that only He knew how to perfectly provide.

The PET scan preparation was more involved than the CT scan. I had to sit in a room for an hour after they injected the nuclear medicine into my bloodstream. I had to remain very still and calm. Because the test will light up sugar, I had nothing to eat prior to the test, only water. It works by attaching itself to any cancer cells and could mistake sugar for cancer cells, lighting them up when the screening is done.

I was asked to sit in a reclining chair in a small dimly lit room. I was told to relax, that this was the longest part of the test. After about an hour, I was told they would come and get me for the actual scan. For now the nuclear medicine would be winding its way through my body.

I knew what I would need to do. I laid back with a warm blanket they provided and turned on my praise and worship music to let the peace of God envelop me. I laid there and worshiped. There was no other way for me to remain calm during this procedure. Once again I needed the presence of the Almighty. It went by relatively quickly. I had the scan and went home.

The next day I got a phone call with the results. It took a while for the words to settle in and for full interpretation to come. The nurse said, "The scan showed no active cancer cells at this time."

No active cancer cells! I was taking it in. I was absorbing this awesomely wonderful news. I was relieved and joyous. After calling Kurt and my mom, I called Rhonda Brown. I had to share this with my overseer's wife and prayer sister. This was a day of celebration.

In the days leading to my surgery date, I wrestled with the question of surgery. Couldn't God just zap the tumors and allow me to escape the process of the surgery? He could do it; I knew He was able. I questioned my faith. Was I not having faith to believe for God to remove the tumors? Was surgery second best to what God had for me in this healing process? These were honest-to-the-core questions for me.

God never minds our questions. He knew I was wrestling over these questions anyway, so I just came out and asked Him and chose not to fear the answer. During my Bible reading (I was reading through the Old Testament), I was working my way through the book of Joshua, and there out of His Word, God spoke to me. It was a very clear and affirmative Word to me and my situation. The Word was this: "By sword or by hailstone."

In Joshua 10 Gibeon had made peace with the children of Israel. They were in alliance with them. So five great kings joined forces to smite Gibeon because of their alliance with Joshua and the children of Israel. The men of Gibeon called on Joshua for help, and Joshua came with all of his mighty men of valor. "And the Lord spoke to Joshua, Fear them not: for I have delivered them into thine hand; there shall not a man of them stand before thee."

The story goes on to share the details of this victory wrought by the hand of God. As I read the story, Joshua 10:11 leaped off the page at me: "And it came to pass, as they fled from before Israel, and were in the going down to Beth-hor-on, that the Lord cast down great stones from heaven upon them unto Azekah, and they died: they were more which died with the hailstones than they whom the children of Israel slew with the sword."

This was my answer to my question. Was surgery a lack of faith on my part? No, it was not. God brings victory in different ways. There were times in this story that Joshua and his mighty men picked up the sword and fought hand to hand. This was not easy for them, but losing was not an option because God was on their side. Other times God sends miraculous, God-timed hailstones to kill the ensuing enemy. But don't be fooled; both victories were by God's hand. He did the work and killed more by the hailstones than by the sword. God used both. The sword and the hailstones were both instruments in His hand, but all the victories, no matter the methodology used, were by His hand.

God was showing me in my healing process that He had already begun a good work in me. His hand was upon me, and the cancer was already dead. This was miraculous in itself, and now God would use surgeons in the next phase of this process. God brings the healing, but it is not for me to say how He will bring it. I would indeed be walking out this process on His terms, knowing that He, the Almighty God, is on my side.

In the waiting period between the end of my chemotherapy treatments and consultation with my team of doctors in Saint

Louis and before my surgeries were to begin, I waited with hope. We continued in prayer, and one night I had a dream.

I have contemplated whether I should share this dream in the book for fear that some may think it a little out there, so to speak. But I have decided it warrants a voice because to me it was a divinely given dream that I believe God used to show me some behind the scenes of what was going on in my situation.

The dream began with a wonderful feeling of my body taking flight. I was accelerating at a high rate of speed upward into the heavenlies. It was a wonderful feeling. I had a tickle in my stomach like you get from riding a roller coaster. I was giggling with laughter. I became aware that someone was with me. I did not know who. We suddenly stopped, and I was standing on an empty, dark planet. Darkness was all around me, there was some light, almost like moonlight but very dim. Someone was holding me by the arm. I looked over behind me and could see what looked like the entrance to a beautiful garden. I could see hanging baskets of flowers. I only glimpsed it. It was as if it was in another place, not the place where I was. There was nothingness where I was standing.

I remember being aware I was in a dream or having a vision, I'm not sure. I thought to myself, "Is that heaven behind me?" I was wondering about the place I had caught a glimpse of. I was not afraid. I looked down at my feet. and the planet beneath me was ash. I remember thinking it looked like volcanic ash. The figure beside me who was holding my arm tugged on me to kneel down. I looked over, and I saw that the figure holding me by the arm was dressed in a hooded cloak. I could not see his face. As we knelt down, I became very aware that I should keep my head down. I was staring at the ash below.

And then there was intense light. It came from behind me and filled the space around me. My focus was no longer the ash but the light. It was so warm, I could feel its warmth going through me. I did not raise my head. There was a sense of godly fear, but I did allow my eyes to look up. The light was going on before me and shone on another place, like a scene from a movie. In it was a young person. It looked as though he was a basketball player, but he was a young person. I could see others but not any others as distinct. And then just like that, the dream was over.

So what did that mean? I did not tell my husband or anyone. I kept it to myself and contemplated the interpretation. I did not have to think about it very long.

Within the next couple of days as I was finishing up reading the Old Testament, I came to a scripture in Malachi 4:2–3 that played out like a scene from my dream: "But unto you that fear my name shall the Sun of righteousness arise with healing in his wings; and ye shall go forth, and grow up as calves of the stall. And ye shall tread down the wicked; for they shall be ashes under the soles of your feet in the day that I shall do this, saith the Lord of hosts."

And then Malachi 4:5–6 continues: "Behold, I will send you Elijah the prophet before the coming of the great and dreadful day of the Lord; And he shall turn the heart of the fathers to the children, and the heart of the children to their fathers, lest I come and smite the earth with a curse."

I believe that in my dream I was caught up before the Lord. Death had me—or maybe it was sickness—but as I stood there the Sun of righteousness arose with healing in his wings. And I believe what I saw beneath my feet were the ashes of my enemies that I had fought in faith and that God had made ashes beneath the soles of my feet. And the next part was to be the next chapter in my life. I had a purpose: to look ahead. The heart of God is to turn the heart of the fathers to the children and the heart of the children to their fathers. I was looking ahead at this young generation.

I decided I would share this with Kurt and with my mother. At first telling they both gasped and felt fear. I knew what they were thinking. They were thinking I was dreaming of dying and going to heaven. But this was not that. When I told them the confirmation that God gave me in scripture, they were wowed by it just as I was.

I'm thankful for this dream and for the continued voice of my Father. I love Him more and more.

Chapter 15

FAITH STEPS

As relived and thankful as I was to be in a position to have surgery, I was also very human. I don't care who you are, knowing that you're going under the knife causes a person to pause and consider life as you know it—not that I hadn't already been doing that in the face of cancer.

Along the way I had listened to a Christian couple testify about the husband's healing of cancer. They told of something they did that I believed was a good idea, and I decided to incorporate it into my journey.

They shared the importance of saying good-bye before the person ever gets to the day of good-bye—basically all those things you really want to say but never do. I really think it is a good idea to do in the face of living not just dying. But so many times we do wait. Why do we wait? Maybe it makes us feel uncomfortable to communicate on that intimate a level. Maybe we feel naked and awkward as we bear our soul to that person, often a beloved family member. I don't know why we do some of the things we do, but we do.

In this couple's testimony, they gave their personal reason for having those intimate, soul-bearing conversations. By sharing these words It freed them from feeling as though they had left something undone or unsaid. It gave them the opportunity to continue to pray in faith for the manifestation of healing, should they choose, without the distraction of feeling they needed to say goodbye. They could instead continue to believe and pray for the fruition of their miracle.

I can only speak to my circumstance. I think you must be very sensitive here to the situation and the desire of the person who is walking through the valley of the shadow of death. I do not forget what scripture says of death in Psalm 116:15: "Precious in the sight of the LORD is the death of his saints."

If as a child of God we sleep in death, we awake with the Father. This is not a dreaded event but a beautiful day of rejoicing for a saint of God. So I don't want to be mistaken here. This world is not our home; it is temporary. Going home to be with our Lord is not a bad thing.

I'm reminded—and please don't be offended—that when we went to China in the early 2000s, we were a bit apprehensive about traveling out of the country for the first time and in a communist country at that. We were concerned about doing anything that might be considered wrong by that culture's standards and putting us and our trip in jeopardy. To lighten the mood, Kurt and I would joke back and forth, "What is the worst thing they can do to us? Send us back to the home of burgers and fries." This was so true. We would just get to go home early.

Forgive the crudeness of the comparison here, but as children of God, when we die—we all will one day if we don't go by way of rapture—then we just get to go home and be with our Heavenly Father. 1 Corinthians 2:9 describes it like this: "But as it is written: 'Eye hath not seen, nor ear heard, neither have entered into the heart of man the things which God hath prepared for them that love Him.'"

Because we believed it was not my time to depart from my earthly home, we chose to press through as a family, doing our best to say what we needed to say prior to surgery. There were tears, laughter, and awkward moments, but we got through it, and I'm glad we did. A sense of relief was associated with it. So let's take a lesson from this and not wait: carpe diem. Tell your loved ones today just what they mean to you. And if there are things to forgive, by all means forgive.

Three weeks later I was checking into the smaller campus of Barnes Jewish for my first surgery. My family and Bishop Tim and Rhonda Brown surrounded me. As pastors ourselves we relied on them as our spiritual shepherds. They arrived at the same time we did that day at the hospital. I can't express how encouraging it is to have a support group that you know is lifting you up in prayer and standing by your side. I did not feel alone, and I could sense the presence of God. The prayers of many were supporting my faith.

The actual colon surgery, done laparoscopically, took less than the estimated time. I was out of surgery in less than two hours. I had eighteen to twenty-four inches of my colon removed. My mom was a little upset that they could not tell us exactly how much was removed, but the doctor did not measure it. In the big scheme of things, it was not so important. He did say that the actual cancerous tumor was nothing more than scar tissue when he removed it. It was also necessary to remove what they called a safe portion on each side of the tumor location in case there were any rogue cancer cells in any of the tissue on either side. He also removed all of the lymph nodes and small blood vessels that led from that portion of my colon to the liver.

The next day I was transferred to the larger campus at Barnes Jewish for the relatively new and innovative portal vein embolization procedure. This procedure was what was making surgery in my case possible and the first step in preparation for the coming liver surgery. During the next four weeks, the healthy portion of my liver would grow and replace itself in size. I am still amazed how God created the human body to do this.

The specialist who could do this procedure worked only at the larger campus. I got to take my first ambulance ride.

During the embolization procedure, no one told us they would also do a liver biopsy. The biopsy was to ensure that my remaining liver was healthy enough to grow. I did not realize the doctors were thinking that because of the twelve chemotherapy treatments, there was a possibility the liver could be damaged. There was, however; no damage—just another opportunity for me to testify of God's keeping power.

I went through the colon surgery with very little pain. In fact I complained more about the embolization done following the colon surgery. I was in the hospital a total of five days and went home on the sixth.

Within two weeks I was walking a mile around the lake at Nathaniel Green Park back in Springfield, and within three weeks I was enjoying a picnic lunch with my daughter there. I found myself on a sure foundation. God was keeping me through surgery and recovery. He was giving me His strength.

This healing time would have to be quick because the second surgery, the liver surgery, would be in five weeks. It was a whirlwind, but God was in it: "Then the LORD answered Job out of the Whirlwind" (Job 38:1).

God will speak to you out of the storm! Listen.

Chapter 16
FAITH FOR THE PUSH

Every finish line has the big push at the end, and I was about to have to find mine. Compared to the colon surgery, this surgery would be no walk in the park. One of the doctor's assistants did tell me, however, that for this doctor, who specialized in liver transplants and pediatric liver transplants to boot, a surgery like mine was a walk in the park. I wanted to remind her that this was my park and no one had ever walked in it. So from my vantage point, it was no walk in the park.

I am laughing here of course. I again am amazed and unbelievably thankful that God had guided me to this place of care. Surely when God moved us from Texas to Missouri some seven years before, He knew even then that I would be facing this cancer diagnosis, and He already had these doctors in place.

So here I was, five weeks and four days after the colon resection and portal vein embolization and headed back to Barnes Jewish Hospital in Saint Louis for the liver lobectomy surgery. Kurt was forever there at my side, supporting me, encouraging me, and basically helping me keep it together. My mom, dad and Zoe had come up for the surgery, and Bishop Brown and his wife, Rhonda were there. Our children, family, and spiritual brothers and sisters from churches everywhere were praying.

We arrived the night before and went for a meal together as a family. I chose my favorite Chinese restaurant. We did not really talk of the surgery; we just enjoyed each other. I did not feel terribly nervous. I was ready to get it over with. We checked into the hotel connected to the hospital and settled in that evening. Yes, we were praying, but we had been praying so we felt secure, safe, and taken care of.

The next morning I had to arrive by five thirty. I am amazed at the attention to detail and the organization that goes into the patient care at these hospitals. I was very well taken care of. I was taken upstairs and prepped. Kurt was with me. An IV was started, and they began to explain to me again what I could expect when I woke up.

I would wake with a nasogastric tube, two IVs just in case something happened to one, a PICC (peripherally inserted central catheter) line into the large vein in my neck, a drain tube in my abdomen, and of course a catheter. I would have two incisions. One would be vertical about five inches in length beginning at the bottom of my breast bone and extending down. The other would be horizontal about twelve inches across the middle of my abdomen. My core was taking a hit. I said good-bye to the abdomen I had known. Not that it was a stellar specimen of abdominal prowess, but however imperfect, it was mine. I would be waking up with an impressive reminder of this storm. I was not feeling vain about what it would look like. I was just thankful that God had made a way for me. And through Jesus Christ, I was more than an overcomer.

Waiting in the bed in pre-op, I looked at the team of doctors standing at my bedside. I was struck by their undivided attention. I was not sure what all this attention meant, but I thought it must mean that this was *really* serious. The doctor, his assistants, the anesthesiologist, and the surgical team were all there talking to me, laughing with me, reassuring me, and answering any last-minute questions to make me feel comfortable. As they talked with me and to each other, I felt the anticipation, the planning, and the preparation that had come down to this moment in time. I was thankful for this team of caring and knowledgeable physicians that God had provided. Most importantly I knew the Great Physician, Jehovah Rapha, and He was with me, orchestrating this whole procedure, infusing His unstoppable, unshakeable power into this situation. His hand was at the helm of my ship in this storm. I knew He would not leave me. Everything was on go. Kurt and I shared a kiss and a prayer before he was asked to leave, and I was rolled down the hall to surgery.

Three hours later I was waking up in ICU. The doctors had explained that as a precaution I would spend the first night in ICU, the second in a step down from that, and the third night in a regular room. Dr. Chapman had come out to speak with my family. I am telling this from their words since I was still in a drug-induced sleep when he reported to them.

He said all went very well. He had removed the right side of my liver. He removed two-thirds. He explained that instead of five tumors, there had been eight. But all were dead tissue and located on the right side where the original five were. He closely examined the remainder of my liver with a sonogram thinking he would find small tumors that the MRI was unable to detect. There were *none*.

He also checked the lymph nodes leading out of my liver. There were *no* signs of cancer cells there. He also said the remainder of the liver was very healthy. There was no bleeding, so no need for a transfusion. He was very pleased. We had prayed specifically for these things.

During my office visit with him prior to the surgery, he had explained he would not be surprised to find small tumors on the left side of my liver and would just burn them out. However, as Kurt and I left his office, I felt in my heart that this would not be the case.

I think I said something like, "I am drawing the line here, and there will not be any tumors in my remaining liver."

My confession was that my liver would be healthy, I would not need a transfusion, and there would be no contamination or infection from the surgery. I was determined and speaking in faith. We called out these specific requests, and God answered everyone.

The first night in ICU Kurt was not allowed to stay with me, although I'm told he spent most of the night in the ICU waiting area. My parents and Zoe stayed in the adjacent hotel.

In the room next to me was some poor woman who was having a difficult time of it. She was yelling at the nurses and refusing to do what they asked her to. It was quite the commotion, so I don't think I slept a lot—but then again maybe I did. I felt no pain and was so very thankful.

The next evening I was ready to be moved to what they call a step-down room from ICU. I had still not sat up. All of the tubes were still running in and out of me. Kurt was with me as they came in and began preparations to move me.

Apparently it was quite an ordeal. Two nurses were attending to me on either side, each one moving quickly and speaking quickly to each other over the top of me. One was going to remove the PICC line, while the other was working on some other part of me. The nurse removing the PICC line explained how important it was for me it was to lie perfectly still as she removed the line and not to lift my head up. She explained the danger of an air bubble going to my brain. OK, momentary panic. I was suddenly not very good. Everything was happening way too fast, and I was feeling overwhelmed and at the mercy of those working quickly around my bedside. I very nicely asked them to back off. They were a bit shocked, and I explained they were going to have to give me a minute, so they should just stop and back away. They did very nicely. They were just doing their job, but it was too much for me at that time.

Kurt came quickly to my side. "Honey, what you need?"

I asked him to read Psalm 91. Very promptly he opened his phone to the Bible app and read Psalm 91 out loud. He knew I was desperate. This was not the first time he had come to my rescue with the Word. There were nights early on in my diagnosis when pain and fear would collide in my body and mind. In the night hours, Kurt would sit beside my bed on the floor, back against the wall, reading the Word of God to me by the light of the headlamp strapped around his head so he would not disturb me with the glare of light.

On this night the nurses stood respectfully over to the side, giving me my needed room. Kurt read the entire chapter, and my angst began to subside. Peace came over me. I just needed to establish by word of mouth whose divine care I was in. I needed to be reminded who was in control: "He who dwells in the secret place of the most High shall abide under the shadow of the almighty. I will say of the Lord He is my refuge and my fortress; my God; in him will I trust" (Psalm 91:1–2).

I was ready now. I told the nurse it was OK to come back over. They were very patient with me. This time I was OK when she removed the PICC line. Trust me, I laid very still.

I was moved to the step-down from ICU, and Kurt was allowed to stay in the room with me that night. The nurse attending to me came in and introduced herself. She wanted to reassure me that she would not do anything to me without asking first and only if it was all right with me. OK, so now I had to be getting a reputation here. I had to be nice.

I said to myself, "Gina, be nice to these people. They are doing their best to take care of you."

I am aware I can be a snarly patient sometimes. Having Kurt in the room with me was a comfort, and I was thankful. I think the nurses were thankful too.

The next day I was doing so well that they moved me to a regular room. They allowed me to sit up in a chair. The tube in my nose was removed, which was a relief. I had not seen the incision yet, but apparently it was something to see. They came often to check on it and make sure that it was healing. Man, oh man, was I sore. I was not in pain. I had some discomfort and soreness, but again they were giving me lots of pain medication. Thank God it worked. Thank God I was not hurting. Thank God the wound was healing. I slept well and had a beautiful view of Saint Louis out of my hospital window, but I was ready to go home.

On the sixth day after surgery, I was released and somewhat apprehensive about the three-and-a-half-hour ride home. I was leaving with instructions to return in four weeks to have the staples removed.

Mom, Dad, and Zoe were waiting for me when I returned home. They were there to help Kurt out in the following weeks. I say help Kurt because he needed it taking care of me. I was a bit whiny after this surgery. I had bounced back so quickly from the colon surgery. I was expecting this to be a little harder, but really I had no idea. The ball was not bouncing very high. In fact it was landing with a thud. Having your core cut makes you extremely sore. Walking, sitting, riding in a car—none of it comes without you knowing it. Your body reminds you with each step.

Nighttime was probably the hardest. I had to sleep with five pillows around me. I would crawl into bed, and Kurt would proceed to tuck the pillows in around me per my instructions. Yes, I was probably bossy and a pain to take care of. I also could not do a lot of personal things without help (I will never be able to repay Kurt for the things he had to do). But little by little, I was getting stronger.

The fourth week I returned to have my staples removed. I was doing very well in keeping with the situation. I did lose weight in the weeks after and during recovery. I did not have a big appetite, and I was uncomfortable. But this weight loss did not hurt me because I had not lost any really to speak of during the chemo or colon surgery.

During this recovery time, there were more days than I would like that I thought I would never get better. And now it was not about being told to rest; it was that I had no choice but to rest. This was not an easy surgery, but I was recovering as scheduled. To pass the time I took up bird watching and am not ashamed to say I rather enjoyed it and still do it today. I continued to rely on the Word and found it to be my daily strength. Kurt and I continued to read Psalm 91 every evening, declaring and establishing by mouth who it was who was protecting and keeping us.

Joel 3:10 says to let the weak say, "I am strong." So each day verbally I would confess, "I am strong." And indeed I was getting stronger.

Chapter 17

FAITH TO MOVE FORWARD

The surgeries were over. The chemotherapy treatments were over. But the impact a serious illness or life event takes on your life and the lives of those you love is forever ingrained in the essence of your existence. Things would never be the same. Life as I knew it had taken a drastic course change. Perspectives had changed. Priorities had been realigned. And now I was having to learn to move forward in this saga of life that I never chose to write. I did not feel like the same person. I was still me but a different version of me.

So how do you move forward? During my first surgery, Caleb and his wife, Ashley, had given birth to our second grandson. Their first son lost his life before it began, and we had buried him in 2013. My oldest son, Aaron, and his wife, Lauren, had given birth a month after my liver surgery to their second beautiful baby girl, adding to their family of three. The fruit of new life was physically manifesting itself all around me. Whether I was ready or not, the world was going to keep turning, the sun would rise and set, and life would go on. I was looking for my new normal. How would I do normal? I couldn't remember.

I found my answer while watching my grandson in early July. Just about seven weeks after my surgery. I was due to go back for a visit with my oncologist. I would still be seeing him for blood work and would continue to have CT scans every three months the remainder of 2015 and 2016. Every time I would go for these visits, I knew full well what they were watching for. They were watching for reoccurrence of cancer, and I would be submitting my faith each time for testing.

I did not like the emotions that I would have to battle before these visits.

I will try and explain. During the course of nine months, I had undergone six months of chemotherapy and two major surgeries. A lot, to say the least, had transpired to me physically as well as mentally, emotionally, and spiritually. I was not in the same place of faith that I had been at the beginning of this journey. My faith in God had become a precious treasure that I had sadly treated with some complacence in the past.

As the day of my oncologist visit approached, I was feeling an internal struggle. I refused to accept fear. After all I had been through, I just wanted to be at ease. I felt as if I was on leave from the front lines of battle, but as I approached the doctor's visit, I found myself having to muster my courage to face the battle, to protect my precious treasure of faith.

But for now I would prepare for Elijah. His parents were bringing him over, and I was looking forward to keeping him for the afternoon.

The morning started as usual. First thing was to take my phone off the nightstand to read the daily scripture. I liked to do this before getting out of bed. The scripture for the day was Jeremiah 32:17: "Alas, Lord God! Behold, You have made the heavens and the earth by your great power and by your outstretched arm! There is nothing too hard for you."

I praised God for this Word; there was nothing too hard for Him. I continued on with my day, getting dressed and preparing to keep Elijah. Shortly thereafter he arrived at my house.

Oh, what a joy it is to watch grandbabies. Besides holding my own children, grandbabies rank right up there at the top of life's most enjoyable and precious blessings. They are a special and miraculous gift from my Heavenly Father, a beautiful fruit of growing older.

Normally Elijah is a laid-back, happy baby with a ready smile, but on this day, he was restless and finding it hard to relax. I tried rocking him, walking with him, and singing and holding him close, but nothing was working. I decided I would lay him down in my bed. I laid him on his side and reached over his little body with my hand and began to pat his little back. I remembered when my children were small patting them until I thought my arm would fall off but not daring to stop because it was lulling them to sleep. As I patted his little back, he seemed to be comforted. His cries turned to small grunts and then just a relaxed sucking of the pacifier. His little body relaxed into the curve of my hand. And then there was the very loud release of what must have been some very uncomfortable trapped gas. Then there was sleep. All was well. Discomfort was gone, replaced by peace and rest.

In that moment I began to hear the quiet, still voice of my Heavenly Father. The morning scripture came back to me. How many times in my life and in the past year had my Heavenly Father reached out His righteous right arm to cradle me, stroke my worried brow, quiet my fearful cries, dry my tears, and, yes, rescue me from the plan of the enemy? A spirit of thankfulness and praise to my precious Heavenly Father overcame me.

During the past year I had faced reports that threatened whether or not I would ever have a moment like today, holding my grandson or any of my grandchildren. But yet here I was, cancer free, enjoying life, a life He had given me.

God saw the mental and emotional roller coaster ride that my nerves were on as I battled for peace in the face of my oncologist visit. But as I continued to look to Him for the answer, He brought it in a very visual, hands-on style. He chose to use a moment with my grandson to speak to me, to remind me that Daddy God is strong and His arm is not too short. Then to further assure me and drive the point home as I sat down for my afternoon devotion, as Elijah was quietly sleeping, this is what I read: "The eternal God is thy refuge, and underneath are the everlasting arms: and he shall thrust out the enemy from before thee; and shall say, Destroy them" (Deuteronomy 33:27).

No, I don't believe it was coincidence. My God is a very present Father. He knows where I am at all times. He knows what I need, and He does not withhold. Then the tears started because the King of the universe, Creator of heaven and earth, cared about me today.

He loves me, this I know.

His arm is outstretched, everlasting and mighty!

My Father had spoken. He was reassuring me as I moved forward in my miracle that His righteous right arm was there to hold me, to keep me. I had nothing to fear because Daddy God was incapable of dropping me.

Almost another year has passed, and my reports continue to come back with no reoccurrence. When speaking with my oncologist and inquiring about my miracle, he concedes that it is indeed a miracle that I could have even had the surgeries. My diagnosis is NED, no evidence of disease.

I continue to walk by faith for each day. I can't have faith for next month or next year. I have faith for today. As it makes sense to continue to let the doctors do their scans, I use it as an opportunity to prove again and again the truth of God's report, by His stripes I was healed. But even more so, it makes sense to me to keep the faith, to guard and protect what I believe and to remember, always, nothing is too hard for God. You are not alone. Do not be afraid. By sword or by hailstone, the Lord is in your victory.

About the Author

Gina Routon, together with her husband, Kurt, have been in full-time ministry with the Church of God for the past twenty-seven years. They currently reside in Mansfield, Texas, where she serves beside Kurt, lead pastor of the Walnut Creek Church. Gina leads the Women's Discipleship Ministries. As a leader and a speaker, her desire is to connect women of all ages to their kingdom purpose by encouraging them to live life authentically in light of God's truth.

www.ingramcontent.com/pod-product-compliance
Lightning Source LLC
Chambersburg PA
CBHW020516290526
45786CB00002B/625